SpringerBriefs in Public Health present concise summaries of cutting-edge research and practical applications from across the entire field of public health, with contributions from medicine, bioethics, health economics, public policy, biostatistics, and sociology.

The focus of the series is to highlight current topics in public health of interest to a global audience, including health care policy; social determinants of health; health issues in developing countries; new research methods; chronic and infectious disease epidemics; and innovative health interventions.

Featuring compact volumes of 50 to 125 pages, the series covers a range of content from professional to academic. Possible volumes in the series may consist of timely reports of state-of-the art analytical techniques, reports from the field, snapshots of hot and/or emerging topics, literature reviews, and in-depth case studies. Both solicited and unsolicited manuscripts are considered for publication in this series.

Briefs are published as part of Springer's eBook collection, with millions of users worldwide. In addition, Briefs are available for individual print and electronic purchase.

Briefs are characterized by fast, global electronic dissemination, standard publishing contracts, easy-to-use manuscript preparation and formatting guidelines, and expedited production schedules. We aim for publication 8–12 weeks after acceptance.

SpringerBriefs in Public Health present concise summaries of cutting-edge research and practical applications from across the entire field of public health, with contributions from medicine, bioethics, health economics, public policy, biostatistics, and sociology.

The focus of the series is to highlight current topics in public health of interest to a global audience, including health care policy; social determinants of health; health issues in developing countries; new research methods; chronic and infectious disease epidemics; and innovative health interventions.

Featuring compact volumes of 50 to 125 pages, the series covers a range of content from professional to academic. Possible volumes in the series may consist of timely reports of state-of-the art analytical techniques, reports from the field, snapshots of hot and/or emerging topics, literature reviews, and in-depth case studies. Both solicited and unsolicited manuscripts are considered for publication in this series.

Briefs are published as part of Springer's eBook collection, with millions of users worldwide. In addition, Briefs are available for individual print and electronic purchase.

Briefs are characterized by fast, global electronic dissemination, standard publishing contracts, easy-to-use manuscript preparation and formatting guidelines, and expedited production schedules. We aim for publication 8–12 weeks after acceptance.

Muyassar Turaeva

Drugs and Public Health in Post-Soviet Central Asia

Soviet-Style Health Management

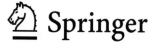 Springer

Muyassar Turaeva
Bielefeld University
Bielefeld, Germany

ISSN 2192-3698   ISSN 2192-3701   (electronic)
SpringerBriefs in Public Health
ISBN 978-3-031-09702-7   ISBN 978-3-031-09703-4   (eBook)
https://doi.org/10.1007/978-3-031-09703-4

This Springer imprint is published by the registered company Springer Nature Switzerland AG
The registered company address is: Gewerbestrasse 11, 6330 Cham, Switzerland

Preface

Soviet-style health governance and the health regimes of authoritarian governments, particularly their punitive measures applied to risky behaviour and epidemiology, is commonly known and well-documented phenomena by now. The most important and relevant institution in this context is the system of *uchyot*, which includes institutions within the fields of medicine, criminal justice and security system, and social and economic fields. The system is made to ensure strong control and apply punitive tools to prevent risky, unwanted and other behaviour leading to epidemiological and other collective risks and problems. Soviet-style biopolitics and health management continue to be practiced in all Central Asian countries. Representative examples of such practices are LTPs (*lechebno-trudovye profilaktorii*, labour correction camps for substance abusers) serving as punitive measures for diverse forms of dependence such as drug and alcohol abuse, among others; psychiatric clinics serving a punitive role within both political and justice systems; venereology and dermatology clinics and departments also serving as punitive institutions for patients with sexually transmitted infections (STIs) and sex workers with or without STIs; narcology clinics playing partly punitive and partly medical roles within the same system of *uchyot* in post-Soviet countries.

The end of Soviet rule came with the collapse of the centralized economy and political transformations in all the Central Asian states. The early post-Soviet years saw declining living standards, weakening public health infrastructure and a decline in life expectancy across most of the Central Asian region. Only Kazakhstan represented a partial exception (Rhodes and Simic 2005[1]). Post-Soviet economic collapse in Central Asia led to accelerated mobility and migration of most labour, mainly to Russia where labourers enjoyed visa-free entrance provided by Post-soviet agreements on economic zones (CIS). Increased mobility, migration, absence of migration policies and labour regulations and the informalization of economies in all the post-Soviet countries led to a devastating public health situation in the region. Authoritarian regimes in most of the post-Soviet countries and particularly in Central Asia and Russia do not allow civil society to develop or effective foreign

---

[1] Transition and the HIV risk environment. *BMJ*. 2005;331:220–3.

aid to address the escalation of current problems, be they medical, health-related, epidemiological, political, economic or social. Authoritarian governments allow little space for addressing health-related problems and don't permit informational enlightenment of the general population to prevent disastrous epidemiological crises, which particularly worsened during and after the COVID-19 pandemic.

In subsequent decades, the public health situation continued to deteriorate, and the system of free health care built by the Soviets has by now completely collapsed (Rechel et al. 2012[2]). The epidemic picture of the region worsened through increased migration, poverty, absence of quality health services and mismanagement at all levels of societal decision-making. Central Asian countries are home to the fastest-growing HIV epidemic in the world, where the main drivers of the epidemic are people who inject drugs (PWIDs) and commercial sex workers (CSWs).

Drug injection and commercial sex work are increasing due to the region's social and economic dislocations and the accompanying psychological stress and alienation, especially among young people. The growing number of people turning to drugs is paralleled by the alarming spread of related diseases such as HIV, hepatitis B and C, and tuberculosis, among other diseases, which make not only particular groups vulnerable to health risks but also the general population.

The COVID-19 pandemic since 2020 not only brought more unnecessary victims suffering as a result of the poor medical infrastructure and capacity but also caused a further dramatic deterioration of the public health situation. Moreover, all Central Asian countries, besides the challenges of the COVID-19 pandemic, further faced problems related to the HIV epidemic, drug abuse and rising rates of hepatitis, tuberculosis, as well as other chronic illnesses, including future long-COVID effects (Smolak et al. 2016[3]; DeHovitz et al. 2014[4]; Donoghoe et al. 2005[5]; Altice 2016[6]). While all countries reported a decline in the supply of traditional drugs, the situation with synthetic drugs is mixed. In Kazakhstan, the number of seizures of synthetic drugs has tripled compared to 2019; in Uzbekistan, the use of pharmaceutical drugs has increased significantly.

This book outlines an institutional setting and behavioural patterns to advance understanding of HIV/AIDS epidemics related to drug abuse in the region, focusing on Uzbekistan. Although the book focuses on a particular context of public health

---

[2] Lessons from two decades of health reform in Central Asia. *Health Policy and Planning.* 2012;27(4):281–7.

[3] Sex workers, condoms, and mobility among men in Uzbekistan: implications for HIV transmission. *International Journal of STD & AIDS.* 2016;27(4):268–72.

[4] The HIV epidemic in Eastern Europe and Central Asia. *Current HIV/AIDS Reports.* 2014;11:168–76.

[5] HIV/AIDS in the transitional countries of Eastern Europe and Central Asia. *Clinical Medicine.* 2005;5:487–90.

[6] The perfect storm: incarceration and the high-risk environment perpetuating transmission of HIV, hepatitis C virus, and tuberculosis in Eastern Europe and Central Asia. *Lancet.* 2016;388(10050):1228–48.

strategies such as post-Soviet countries, it will still be contextualized within the global fight against HIV and drug abuse.

The book is based on qualitative study, where the empirical data were collected during long-term fieldwork conducted in Uzbekistan in 2010–2011 as well as shorter stays between 2012 and 2016. The qualitative methods used included semi-structured interviews, group discussions, participant observations, clinical observations, autobiographies and informal conversations. All names and other personal identifiers of informants included in the book have been changed to protect their privacy and confidentiality. The data and material collected for this book were analysed using a theoretical framework offered by the works of Michel Foucault on biopolitics, which is particularly relevant for the study of Soviet-style health governance. Applying a Foucauldian genealogical method, the study is structured to trace the genealogy of epidemics to understand the historical path of drug abuse in the region as well as the discursive genealogy of drug politics and drug abuse. Applying the same genealogical method of Foucault, the formative and discursive trajectory of the institution of *uchyot* was traced to contextualize the health governance methods which have a historical legacy of Soviet-style governance and control over the general population.

The book offers not only important in-depth insights into current and past developments of the public health situation in post-Soviet Central Asia but also contributes further to analytical and theoretical advancements, presenting the empirical realities of Foucauldian biopolitics and Soviet-style health management. This analysis suggests further opportunities for the advancement of a Foucauldian approach within the public health studies in post-Soviet countries (Turaeva and Turaeva 2021[7]). The book also offers recommendations for both international and national actors who are active in the region studying and addressing the problems analysed in the chapters.

This book offers in-depth reflections on the institutional infrastructure in place to manage the HIV/AIDS epidemic related to drug abuse in Uzbekistan, highlighting how this epidemic evolved and how it is now governed (biopolitics). Moreover, the book will further outline behavioural patterns of drug abuse focusing on the role of these patterns in the dynamics of the epidemics to be able to show the links between HIV/AIDS, drug abuse and mobility. Finally, the book addresses such questions as whether these interdependencies influence the general dynamics of the epidemic and what factors contribute to the risky behaviour of drug users.

The main argument of this book is that the Soviet style of (mis)management of disease and an iron-handed approach to at-risk groups pushes such groups into the shadows of survival and contributes to additional risks. In the case of drug users, additional risks include secret drug injections made in unsanitary conditions and with used equipment. Information-sharing takes place from peer to peer to avoid contact with the state or other official sources of medical information. Secrecy and the fear of being detected and listed in state semi-official registers (*uchyot*)

---

[7] *Uchyot* and Foucault: drug users and migration in Uzbekistan. *Central Asian Affairs*. 2021;8:83–98.

contributed to the outbreak of epidemics in these countries (Turaeva and Turaeva 2021). Furthermore, other factors such as social status and gender, as well as economic situation and mobility, I argue, are also important in explaining the behaviour of drug users.

Special attention is also given to female drug users both with and without HIV infection. I detail different life circumstances and show the vulnerability of female PWIDs to violence (from sexual partners, police and family members) and to stigmatization (by society and family), both of which contribute to an increased risk of exposure to HIV. Gender roles and labour distribution with respect to both drug consumption and sex work are determined by general patriarchal social norms which place female drug users and sex workers in the weakest economic positions, impose on them the greatest labour burdens within families, and leave them to face burdensome responsibilities and social pressures. In a patriarchal society, it is difficult enough to be a woman; to be in addition a drug user causes women to slip through already limited networks of social support and solidarity (not to mention the state system of health care and social support). The incorrect beliefs held by female drug users about infectious diseases make them yet more vulnerable to unprotected sex.

Furthermore, I argue that the shift in patterns of drug use (from smoking to injection) in the region due to a lack of knowledge about drugs among the general population, huge inflow of heroin to Uzbekistan from Afghanistan (new developments in the region are still to be seen under the Taliban), the restriction of 'traditional drugs' and further tightening of control over drug use, and the sudden disruption of drug inflow has been a crucial development contributing to the outbreak of diseases such as HIV. This, coupled with a collapsing healthcare system, poor investments in hygiene and public health, and unprofessional medical personnel, led to a devastating epidemic crisis in the region, escalating with the current COVID-19 pandemic (Coreil 2001[8]; UNODC 2020[9]).

The book not only offers important in-depth insights into current and past developments of the public health situation in post-Soviet Central Asia but also contributes further to analytical and theoretical advancements, showing the empirical realities of Foucauldian biopolitics and Soviet-style health management. The analysis presented in the book suggests further opportunities for the advancement of the Foucauldian approach to public health studies in post-Soviet countries (Turaeva and Turaeva 2021). The book also offers recommendations for both international and national actors active in the region studying and addressing the problems analysed in the chapters.

Bielefeld, Germany   Muyassar Turaeva

---

[8] *Social and Behavioral Foundations of Public Health.* Library of Congress. 2001.

[9] Brief overview of COVID-19 impact on the drug use situation as well as on the operations of drug treatment services and harm reduction programmes in Central Asia. 2020. https://www.unodc.org/documents/centralasia/2020/August/3.08/COVID-19_impact_on_drug_use_in_Central_Asia_en.pdf.

Acknowledgments

This work is dedicated to my daughter Paulina and other family members who were always there to help, support, understand, advise, help, and care about me and my work without whom this work would have been impossible.

I sincerely would like to thank my family without whose support this research and eventually the book would not be possible. My sincere gratitude goes to Rano Turaeva (my sister) and Markus Hoehne who supported my fieldwork financially and further supported my work throughout the uneasy long path out of which this book also came to light. Their anthropological influence in my methodology and further in my analysis was valuable for this research. Other members of my big family was important therefore I thank my parents Djanil Amanova and Atadjan Turaev, my sisters Muhabbat Turaeva, Mamura Turaeva, Ugiljon Turaeva, as well as other members such as Feruza and Steven Obsts.

This book is based on the invaluable information entrusted to me by my informants during my fieldwork in Uzbekistan and Turkmenistan and afterwards, some of whom continue to the present to maintain contact with me; without their trust, this book would not have been possible. I deeply appreciate their help and their direct contribution to my work throughout my research.

Furthermore I thank Prof. Dr. Ralf E. Ulrich, who served as a supervisor of this doctoral research on which this book is based upon.

I am also very grateful to my friends Min and Katarina Rost who supported me cheerfully.

Contents

About the Author

Muyassar Turaeva, PhD is a public health scientist. She obtained her Master's in Public Health from Charité University of Medicine and PhD in Public Health from Bielefeld University, both located in Germany. Her mainly research activities focus on gender, health, drug addiction, HIV and near-death experiencex, and her research findings have been published in journals such as *Kultur und Gesellschaft Opladen*, *Journal of Substance Use*, *Advanced Studies in Medical Sciences*, and *British Journal of Applied Science & Technology*.

List of Acronyms

ART	Antiretroviral treatment
CADAP	Central Asia Drug Action Programme
CAR	Central Asian Republic
CDC	Centers for Disease Control and Prevention (USA)
CSW	Commercial sex worker
EMCDDA	European Monitoring Centre for Drugs and Drug Addiction
HBV	Hepatitis B virus
HCV	Hepatitis C virus
HIV/AIDS	Human immunodeficiency virus/acquired immunodeficiency syndrome
IHRD	Institute of Human Resources Development
IISS	International Institute for Strategic Studies
INCSR	International Narcotics Control Strategy Report
MSM	Men who have sex with men
NEP	Needle exchange programme
PWIDs	People who inject drugs
STI	Sexually transmitted infection
TB	Tuberculosis
UNAIDS	Joint United Nations Programme on HIV/AIDS
UNDP	United Nations Development Programme
UNODC	UN Office for Drug Control and Crime Prevention
USAID	United States Agency for International Development
USSR	Union of Soviet Socialist Republics
WHO	World Health Organization

List of Figures

List of Tables

Uzbek PWID Slang

bayan, mashinka	syringe
butor	diluted heroin, something added to heroin to increase the amount
chek, kichkina	unit of measurement for powdery drug
dimka, dimyan, dima	Dimedrol
gera, ok, shakar, un, haydar, karim, vaj, vasevka	heroin
gref	invitation for drugs (or service) free of charge
gvozd/mih, shtiket, idish, belomorka, nasha, anasha, haydar, korobok, kuk choy	cannabis
jaruyha	porridge from cannabis
kasal, humor	withdrawal symptoms
kora dori, kora, hanka, kora choy, lya [ля ля]	opium
kosyak	cigarette filled with drugs (usually with cannabis)
kotur	mixed heroin
maymul	smart
musora	police
narsa, vaj	drugs
pulesos	person who sniffs heroin
remashka	relanium
shirovy, shirik	low-class intravenous drug user
tochka	place where one can buy heroin
tonna	1 gram of heroin
veshdok	evidence
vmazuvatsya	inject drugs
vybiraesh	sucking into syringe
yarim tonna	0.5 gram heroin

Chapter 1
Introduction

1.1 Drug Abuse and Public Health in Central Asia

What happens when states continuously try to suppress, oppress, control and manage unwanted behaviour and force healthy lifestyles is the main question this book will try to address. It will also offer in-depth insights into the lives of drug users, sex workers, people with HIV and those who were marked and labeled as unwanted and denied any kind of support to survive. I partly detail in this book the stark means these individuals use to somehow survive the hardships of being physically and mentally unwanted, where no numbers can show their misery.

In Central Asian countries with the highest incidence rates of new HIV cases over the last decade, with 100,000 new HIV infections in 2019 alone (UNAIDS 2019a), the main drivers of the epidemic were people who inject drugs (PWIDs), their sexual partners, commercial sex workers (CSWs), men who have sex with men (MSM) and prisoners (UNAIDS 2019b). Central Asia, as it is used in this book, includes five countries: Uzbekistan (33,469,203), the Kyrgyz Republic (6,524,195), Tajikistan (9,537,645), Turkmenistan (6,031,200) and Kazakhstan (18,776,707), with a total population of more than 60 million culturally, ethnically and religiously diverse people. The most recent population size estimates show that there are 42,425 PWIDs in 2019 in Uzbekistan (UNDAF 2019), 120,500 in Kazakhstan (UNAIDS 2016), 25,000 in the Kyrgyz Republic (UNAIDS 2016) and 25,000 in Tajikistan (EMCDDA 2014a, b); no data exist for Turkmenistan. There are no reliable long-range epidemiological data on drug use in Central Asia.

Drug injection and commercial sex are increasing due to the region's social and economic dislocations and the accompanying psychological stress and alienation, especially among young people. The growing number of people turning to drugs parallels the alarming spread of related diseases such as HIV, hepatitis B and hepatitis C virus (HCV). Injection drug use in the WHO-defined Eastern European and Central Asia (EECA) is among the highest in the world, with a prevalence of 0.63%

M. Turaeva, *Drugs and Public Health in Post-Soviet Central Asia*,
SpringerBriefs in Public Health, https://doi.org/10.1007/978-3-031-09703-4_1

in Central Asia (Degenhardt et al. 2017). Globally, drug abuse and health are treated in an interdisciplinary manner using diverse approaches (Leshner 1997; Vrecko 2006; Campbell 2007; Valverde 1998). Globally, in terms of the problem of injection drug abuse, it is estimated that there are 15.9 million people who inject drugs (between 11 and 21.2 million) (Mathers et al. 2010). Eastern Europe (1.5%) and Australia and New Zealand (1.03%) have a high prevalence of injection drug abuse. In absolute numbers, Eastern Europe has one of the highest numbers of injecting drug users. In Eastern Europe most of the injecting users use opiates, while in Australia and New Zealand, methamphetamine is the main substance being injected. Central Asia stands in the middle in terms of ranking. Most of the literature on drug abuse is largely based on examples from Latin America, Eastern Europe and Southeast Asia. The literature on drug abuse in Eastern Europe focuses on drug policies, medication-assisted treatment (MAT), drug treatment and harm reduction (LaMonaca et al. 2019; Stoever et al. 2020; Vranken et al. 2017). The same scholarship on similar issues on Central Asia is largely treated within the group of Eastern Europe or Asian regions. The post-Soviet context offers a much more historically and politically relevant context which needs to be considered separately as such a designation of the analysis within the wider geographic context runs a risk of underestimating some of the relevant particularities. Moreover, one needs to pay more attention to the recent history of the same region, namely the Soviet past. This aspect is of particular importance when looking at most of the post-Soviet countries, which is one of the most important contributions of this book.

The collapse of the Soviet centralized economy and post-Soviet political transformations in all Central Asian states had grave implications for the general situation of public health in the region. The early post-Soviet years saw declining living standards, weakening public health infrastructure and declines in life expectancy across most of the Central Asian region. Only Kazakhstan constituted a partial exception (Rhodes and Simic 2005; Ancker and Rechel 2015). The later post-Soviet period did not improve but rather the situation of public health continued to deteriorate without the replacement of the old Soviet system of health management (Rechel et al. 2012a, 2013; McKee et al. 2014). In terms of the prevalence of drug use, officially registered consumption is decreasing slightly (especially in Kazakhstan and Uzbekistan and among newly registered persons). Newly registered HIV infections, the proportion of injecting drug users in all Central Asian countries, is decreasing, possibly due to existing syringe exchange programmes (Michels et al. 2021). Based on a report released by the United Nations Development Assistance Framework (UNDAF) (2021), indicators show decreasing trends in the numbers of registered (5857 in 2019 against 6291 in 2018) and treated drug users.

Public health problems reaching critical levels have caught the attention of scholars who analyse the outbreak of HIV epidemics, drug abuse and the rising rates of hepatitis as well as other chronic illnesses (Smolak et al. 2016; DeHovitz et al. 2014; Donoghoe et al. 2005; Platt et al. 2020; Baillargeon et al. 2017). These developments in the region can also be partly explained through structural, societal, behavioural and other changes associated with a new political and economic reality following the collapse of the Soviet Union and later by the mismanagement of economies and bad governance (Kupatadze 2012).

1.2   (Mis)management of Public Health in Central Asia

In developed economies, health care is organized in terms of providing care for those who face health problems and those who need support for their well-being, whereas in other countries or regions, such as in the post-Soviet context, health is managed and controlled. This has a major impact not only on the epidemiological situation in the region but also on the general well-being of all individuals. Healthcare provisions in each context need to consider not only the general principles of healthcare provision but also be receptive to cultural aspects of individual attitudes towards well-being and knowledge about healthy lifestyles.

(Mis)management of public health and general healthcare governance has a particular political and historical background in Central Asia. I consciously use the word 'management' instead of 'care' when discussing healthcare delivery systems or issues related to governance and administration within the system of health care. The aim of the strategic use of these terms is to underline the approach to population rather than individual health and choice to manage rather than care for the health and individual well-being of each resident in a given country. Soviet-style health management and strict control of the population's health is a dominating principle used by most post-Soviet or ex-Soviet republics today and were also striking features evident during the health crisis of the COVID-19 pandemic (Antonov and Edward 2021). Burkle (2020) argued that autocratic regimes define public health policies along economic and political imperatives, which is largely observed in many countries with similar political regimes. Autocratic regimes tend to undermine the health consequences of infectious diseases or their impacts on populations, as is also largely observed in Central Asia, where the governments are quick to sacrifice the lives of citizens for personal gain or in service to a personality cult (e.g. Turkmenistan ignoring the COVID virus at the cost of many countless lives). Burkle (2020) gives examples of authoritarian regimes. Authoritarian regimes in China, Russia, North Korea and some African countries, where ruling elites pursue their personal agendas at times not necessarily good for general populations particularly in the issues concerning public health or social wellfare. At times the authoritarian goverments fail to follow recommendations which would require state actions to prevent health crisis or public health problems, taking timely precautions, deny accurate scientific conclusions that contradict facts, their wishes and do not meet the health expectations for public health under existing international health regulations, laws and surveillance.

Although Central Asian republics took varying political paths following the break-up of the Soviet Union, they share several public health issues. Public health problems shared by all Central Asian republics include HIV/AIDS outbreaks, hepatitis, tuberculosis (TB), sexually transmitted infections (STIs), drug abuse and other chronic illnesses. These problems are commonly found in contexts where poverty and a lack of state social provisions and political insecurities prevail. The same problems are addressed differently in other countries, such as in Belarus and Russia (Lundgren et al. 2014).

Central Asian governments have also addressed the same problems differently depending on their political and economic conditions, which also depended on the path taken by each Central Asian individual government, and those paths differed in form but were largely similar in content (for instance renaming LTPs (labour correction camps for substance abusers)s but keeping the same practices in other forms).[1] The national response of the Uzbek government to the outbreak of HIV and drug abuse was reflected in the work of state healthcare institutions, narcology clinics, AIDS clinics and derma-venereology dispensaries. Some funding was made available also for non-governmental orgaizations (NGOs), and the mass media was asked to get involved in promoting healthy lifestyles and in informing the public about drug abuse and its consequences. The Tajik government, for instance, chose a violent way of addressing the rise of HIV infection by criminalizing it, which directly violates human rights to sexual health for all persons living with HIV. According to the legal amendments, persons living with HIV are not permitted to have sex following the Article 125 of the Criminal Code of Tajikistan. When a criminal case is initiated under this article, the status of both the suspect and the victim is simultaneously disclosed. The legislation does not consider exceptions in connection with the informed consent of the other sexual partner (regardless of whether there was the risk of HIV infection) or whether the virus carrier is taking precautions like wearing a condom (Alexandrova 2021). The Turkmen government, during the presidency of former president Niyazov, reduced the healthcare infrastructure (Peyrouse 2019) under the motto 'our nation is a healthy nation', which also led to a reduction of personnel, leading to a major public health disaster in the country. This shortage of personnel and healthcare infrastructure played out during the pandemic, which is also shamefully ignored by the current president under the motto 'we are the best nation with zero COVID cases'. Since 2022, the son of the president of Turkmenistan took over the presidency, continuing his father's legacy, and is notorious for his brutality.[2] The COVID disaster of the delta variant is unfolding at the time of this writing, giving rise to an unknown but high number of deaths in the country. In the same vein, over the past 20 years, Turkmenistan has not reported cases of HIV infection, but at the same time, 113 and 10 Turkmen citizens with HIV were identified and registered in Russia and Kazakhstan respectively.[3] The Kazakh and Kyrgyz governments followed a generally more liberal approach politically and economically, opening their economies and more or less following the principles of democratic governance (Kukeyeva and Shkapyak 2013) to orient their countries to the West. In these two Central Asian countries, the Western influence, such as American and European principles of economic and political reform, was felt more than in Uzbekistan, Tajikistan or Turkmenistan. Although the Central Asian countries took their own path in reforming or not reforming their Soviet-era healthcare systems,

---

[1] I describe LTPs in this book in a more detailed manner; it is an important institution which was a punitive structure for substance abusers in the Soviet Union.

[2] The first things the new president of Turkmenistan introduced in 2022 was prohibiting beauty services for women under the motto 'women are naturally beautiful and do not need these services'. Personal communication with relatives, April 20, 2022.

[3] Technical Workshop on HIV and Migration for Central Asian Countries and the Russian Federation 19–20 February 2018. https://afew.org/wp-content/uploads/2019/11/HIV-REPORT_RUS_FIN_1.pdf.

they all share a common history and comparable cultural and traditional patterns of understanding human well-being and health, and most of the countries have largely remained authoritarian regimes (Kupatadze 2012).

In the national plan for combating HIV/AIDS, one could follow the trace of the still Soviet style of health management with strategies that read as follows: 'To integrate HIV/AIDS/STI problems into the key concepts of the Republic of Uzbekistan's development, through multi-sectoral collaboration' (Godinho et al. 2005). Multi-sectoral collaboration in the local context would mean more sharing of data among medical, security and other areas of state and society relations, not in a positive sense, which it might initially sound like, but rather in the sense of greater collaborative control over unwanted behaviour.

Uzbekistan is a signatory to a range of international conventions. In the same year, Uzbekistan signed the Central Asian Counternarcotics Memorandum of Understanding with the United Nations Office on Drugs and Crime UNODC and agreed to the establishment of a Central Asian Regional Information and Coordination Centre (CARICC) to coordinate information sharing and joint counternarcotics efforts in Central Asia. Although the EU Central Asia Drug Action Programme (CADAP) stands out among other international programmes against drug abuse and other health-related problems, there are significant gaps in the ways the programme reaches out to the target group due to the problems I detail in this book (Zabransky and Mravcik 2019). The same can be said of capacity-building activities which need a more systematic and more engaging approach to achieve the aims set out within the programme. Gaining trust is the most important and most challenging aspect of any initiative addressing vulnerable populations such as drug users. There have been important publications resulting from the project's activities, which contribute to the gaps in the field, which remains understudied (Michels et al. 2017; Stoever et al. 2016, 2019, 2020).

According to Stoever et al. (2016), harsh criminal sanctions were imposed on PWIDs, resulting in escalating incarceration rates, especially of those who either had or were at high risk for HIV. Additionally, against a backdrop of economic instability and low salaries of the police, these individuals became targets for bribes and other forms of corruption. An inability to pay resulted in arrests, detention and imprisonment, which my findings also support. Other sources (Stone and Shirley-Beavan 2018; Stoever 2010; Altice et al. 2016) indicate a high risk of contracting infectious diseases, such as hepatitis, TB and HIV, in prison settings. Soviet-style health management largely remains as the model of healthcare delivery and healthcare management in Central Asia, despite a decade of involvement of international assistance programmes. Soviet-style health care was initially formulated according to the visions and perspectives developed by Prof. Semashko, who is the main author of the various Soviet healthcare models, and the whole system was named after him: the Semashko system of health care. This system is characterized by overcentralized healthcare delivery available for free to all citizens. However, the same system gives greater priority to infectious diseases than non-infectious ones.

The most important continuity of healthcare administration from the Soviet period is the system of cooperation between medical, security and other state institutions to control health risks and outbreaks. This system has no medical ethics, for instance, patient anonymity, security of medical data, security of identity or other issues related to morality and ethics. The system of control over unwanted behaviour, such as drug abuse, prostitution, criminal activity or anything else considered harmful to society, is known under the name of *Uchyot* (literally from the Russian for 'registration' and meaning *blacklisting*) (Turaeva and Turaeva 2021). Such a system of control of people's health and bodies resembles the principles of biopolitics described by Foucault (1997). The *Uchyot* system is used to prevent risky and unwanted behaviour that may lead to epidemiological and other collective risks. This system, which attempts to control the public health situation by managing bodies and intervening in the private lives of individuals who might engage in risky behaviour, can be explained by applying analytical tools based on the biopolitical principles of governance defined by Michel Foucault. His concept of biopolitics in particular is useful here. If an individual wants to move, which is also undesirable in the eyes of the authorities, he or she must deal with the system of residence registration (*propiska*), which is restrictive both in Russia and in Central Asia (Turaeva & Urinboyev 2021).

1.3 Drug Trafficking Routes in Central Asia

The Taliban's rise to power in Afghanistan (as of August 2021) will have major security and political implications in Central Asia, which is considerable for the general epidemiological situation in Central Asia. These and other developments in the region (the war in Ukraine, the COVID-19 crisis, the economic crisis following both of these events and the sanctions against Russia) make the region particularly vulnerable politically, economically and socially. Drug-trafficking routes are another issue to consider when analysing drug abuse and the availability of drugs in the region. The world's use of heroin and cocaine has been on an upward trend since the early 1990s (Storti and Grauwe 2009). Globally, 11 million people inject drugs (Mathers et al. 2008; WHO 2021). The cultivation of opium poppy was widespread in parts of Russia, Ukraine, Uzbekistan and Kazakhstan (Dehne et al. 1999). However, the heroin in global circulation is produced in three regions of the world, Southwest Asia (Afghanistan), Southeast Asia (Myanmar, Laos) and Latin America (Colombia and Mexico). Of these, the bulk of heroin comes from Afghanistan; in 2007 it produced more than 90% of the world's opiates (IHRD 2008). The production of cocaine is prevalent in Bolivia, Colombia and Peru. The marketing route of heroin crosses Central Asian countries to reach users in Russia and Europe. After the break-up of the Soviet Union, the new borders remained poorly administered, and national customs services were created only by 1993–1994 (Brill et al. 2000). This facilitated the formation of a northern drug trafficking route from Afghanistan through Central Asia – a 'second golden triangle' (IISS 1997; Zabransky et al. 2014). The route runs through Uzbekistan to Tajikistan. The rise to power of the Taliban in Afghanistan in 2021 will have further implications for drug-trafficking and drug-consumption patterns in the region.

The expansion of drug use followed: UNODC (2010) reported 283,000 heroin users in Central Asian countries. Moreover, Godinho et al. (2005) showed that the drug industry has become deeply embedded within local economies. In Tajikistan, drug trafficking contributed to almost half of the country's national income. Research findings by Kupatadze (2014) on the involvement of politicians and police officials in criminal activities support the argument that key income-generating activity in Kyrgyzstan involves law enforcement officials, who have gradually become embroiled in illegal business and over time have carved out their own market share in the drug trade (the findings cover the period of Bakiev's presidency).

Afghan heroin production has skyrocketed since 2000 and has further impacted the health of local populations along the drug route. According to estimations of UNODC, 99% of opiates in CA originate from Afghanistan (UNODC 2008b). The latest available figures from INCB (2020) indicated that the amount of heroin seized in Kazakhstan, Kyrgyzstan, Tajikistan, Turkmenistan and Uzbekistan increased by 69.6% in 2019 compared with 2018, whereas the amount of opium seized decreased by 41.3%. In total, 5.7 tons of opiates were seized in 2019, compared with 5.3 tons in 2018. The disturbing level of opium consumption in the countries bordering Afghanistan (Uzbekistan, Turkmenistan, Tajikistan, Pakistan, Iran) was estimated at 6500 metric tons per year, which constituted 60% of global consumption (UN 2018; UNODC 2010). It is also important to note that 25% of the total export of Afghan heroin is consumed in Central Asian countries (about 100 tons) (UNODC 2009:11). According to UNODC (2010: 49), drugs mainly penetrate Uzbekistan through Tajikistan because Uzbekistan's borders with Afghanistan are well policed. However, complex geographical conditions in the Termez region led to the development of porous 'windows' through which Afghan drugs penetrate and further spread to Karshi, Bukhara, Urgench and Nukus (Hohlov 2006). The Khorezm region had a high number of registered opiate users, and the Surkhandarya district (bordering Afghanistan and Tajikistan), Jizzak (bordering Tajikistan) and Samarkand also have a high number of drug users (UNODC 2008b). Most opiate shipments are trafficked through Uzbekistan along the south-east/north-west axis (along the M-37 Samarkand-Navoi-Bukhara highway, or along the A-380 Karshi-Bukhara-Nukus highway) through western Kazakhstan into the Russian Federation (UNODC 2018). UNODC (2008a) estimates that as many as 130,000 people, or 0.8% of the total adult population (15–64 years), were dependent on opiates. In Tashkent alone, 1.2% of the adult population, or 16,000 people, were dependent on opiates (ibid). An alarming development is that the total global opium production jumped to 10,500 tons in 2017, the highest estimate recorded by UNODC since it started monitoring global opium production in the early twenty-first century (UNODC 2018).

In 2020, Deputy Minister of Internal Affairs Azizbek Ikramov said that 5889 young citizens had been registered as drug users in Uzbekistan. Most of these drug user citizens are registered in the Andijan region – 1232 people, the Fergana region – 1093, and Tashkent – 1188.[4] The reliance on the national statistics is unavoidable, although national statistics and the reporting system on health care is suspect

---

[4] Gazeta.uz; https://www.gazeta.uz/ru/2020/09/11/narcotic/.

because of the outdated methodology of data collection and the general attitude of drug users, who avoid registration and health officials. Reports by international projects showed that the situation with drug abuse saw considerable numerical improvement, but there remains a large gap and more qualitative, systematic, basic research needs to be performed in order to be able to address the problems related to drug abuse and HIV/AIDS in the region. Reported trends in drug abuse in Uzbekistan have improved slightly (Michels et al. 2017), which was explained as being the result of several large-scale initiatives, such as a multi-phase border management programme in Central Asia (BOMCA) and CADAP, which are found in the reports of the same CADAP programme (Zabransky and Mravcik 2019). Independent monitoring and systematic studies are needed to prove the viability of this trend in order to draw valid conclusions about such reports.

Drug trafficking via Central Asian states became more challenging during the COVID-19 pandemic owing to the closure of state borders and the resulting restrictions on the movement of people and goods. This might have weakened the ability of organized criminal groups to smuggle drugs, but the risk of opiate trafficking continued to exist, as commercial cargo and food products continued to be transported (INCB 2020). Due to COVID-19-related restrictions, different impacts on the supply and demand of drugs have been observed in the region. In Kazakhstan, Kyrgyzstan, Tajikistan and Turkmenistan, quantities of opiates seized declined during the first half of 2020 compared with the same period in 2019; this development was attributed to a reduction in supply. In Kazakhstan trafficking groups have actively tried to organize the illicit manufacture of synthetic drugs within the country (World Drug Report 2021). The findings of CARICC (2020) show links to existing drug-trafficking routes, migration and drug dependence rates in the region. There is ample evidence that the establishment of a drug-trafficking route through Central Asia influenced drug use patterns in the region, changing them from a 'traditional' way of smoking opium to a risky drug consumption pattern (injecting) and, consequently, the escalation of the HIV epidemic in the region (UNODC 2008b). International organizations reported early on (UNDP 2008; UNODC 2008b) that there was a relationship between the drug route and high HIV prevalence in Uzbekistan, where the numbers were high in certain locations located along drug-trafficking routes. These are the city of Tashkent, Tashkent oblast, Surkhadarya, Samarkand and Fergana oblast in Uzbekistan. Tashkent is the capital city of Uzbekistan, where most HIV cases are concentrated (76% of all cases), fueled by a high rural-to-urban migration flow (UNDP 2008). The same pattern of concentration of HIV cases in regions located along trafficking routes generally for Central Asia is also observed: in Kazakhstan, in the districts of Karaganda, the city of Almaty, Zhambyl province; in Kyrgyzstan, the urban centres of Bishkek, the city of Osh and Chui oblasts; in Tajikistan, the capital city of Dushanbe and Gorno-Badakhshan Autonomous District.

1.4   HIV Epidemics in Central Asia and Migration

HIV is transmitted through contact with infected blood and bodily fluids. Such contact can occur through unprotected sex, through sharing needles or other drug injection paraphernalia, through mother-to-child transmission during pregnancy or breastfeeding, and through infected blood transfusions and plasma products. While effective antiretroviral therapy (ART) is available, there is currently no cure for HIV/AIDS (Archin and Margolis 2014; Barton et al. 2013). According to recent data provided by UNAIDS (2019c), HIV is still prevalent among PWIDs, who account for 5.1% of the 5400 total HIV respondents from 2018 (Table 1.1). The situation of HIV infection before 2015 was not much different from the current situation. The HIV epidemic was mainly concentrated among PWIDs in Central Asia before 2015 (IHRD 2008). The higher share of HIV transmission is attributed to drug injection as the predominant mode of transmission, for example 73.6% in Kazakhstan, 75% in Kyrgyzstan and 60% in Uzbekistan. Transmission through non-sterile medical equipment and blood transfusions remains unclear as there is no systematic observation of these practices, and evidence for such incidents is simply anecdotal (Lillis 2012; Mirovalev 2010; Baigin and Humphries 2010; Vennard 2008). These practices are not, of course, reported and victims either remain silent or do not have enough information about transmission methods and consequences of such an infection.

According to UNAIDS estimations, drug abuse remains the most prevalent group among HIV-infected persons, although the hidden numbers can be different in light of the COVID crisis, where migrants working in Russia had been forced to return back to Uzbekistan. Based on a UNAIDS report (2019c), HIV prevalence since 2015 has increased slightly (Table 1.2).

Uzbekistan has an estimated HIV prevalence of 0.15% (52,000 cases) among the general population. In 2018, the Joint United Nations Programme on HIV/AIDS (UNAIDS) estimated that there were 16 cases of HIV per 100,000 adult population in the country (UNAIDS Data 2018). UNDAF (2021) reported that in Uzbekistan there were 3983 new HIV cases in 2019 (4060 in 2018). The proportion of PWIDs

Table 1.1   Key population

	Sex workers	Gay men and MSM	PWIDs	Prisoners
HIV prevalence	3.2%	3.7%	5.1%	0.5%

Statistical data sourced from UNAIDS (2019c)

Table 1.2   Epidemic estimates

	2010	2015	2018
New HIV infections	4100	500	5400
HIV prevalence (15–49)	[0.1]	[0.2]	[0.2]

Statistical data sourced from UNAIDS (2019c)

among people living with HIV (PLHIV) is decreasing. In 2019, this number was 42,425 (40,376 in 2018). PLHIV were registered in the country, of whom PWIDs made up 4842 or 11.41%. The statistical data on Uzbekistan shows alarming patterns of speed of transmission, equal distribution among sexes and the fact of increasing numbers of HIV infection among pregnant women, which has further implications for prenatal health care.

Before 2015, during fieldwork statistical information on HIV and drug abuse was not much different from the current statistics outlined above. According to Mounier et al. (2006), the Central Asian countries are following the same epidemiological pattern of HIV epidemic and have trajectories similar to those in Russia and Ukraine. The outbreak of HIV and STI epidemics in Central Asia began in the early 1990s, coinciding with the collapse of the Soviet Union. The first five cases of HIV infection were recorded in 1987 in Uzbekistan (Zhao et al. 2020) among foreign students from Africa. Before the 2000s, little was known about HIV in Uzbekistan (ibid 2020). By 2001, the recorded incidence rose to 800. In 2006 alone, 2205 new HIV cases were recorded (UNODC 2008a, b: 34). Once HIV infection entered Uzbekistan, PWIDs became a source of both parenteral and sexual transmission of HIV infection in the republic. For years, the epidemic was mainly concentrated among PWIDs, but since 2010 sexual transmission has become the predominant mode of transmission (Zhao et al. 2020). Research conducted in Uzbekistan (1987–2002) in collaboration with an AIDS clinic investigated the molecular epidemiology of HIV (Kurbanov et al. 2003). A total of 18,910,370 subjects were screened through a population survey, and genetic subtype A and 03_CRF-A/B variants of HIV infection were identified among PWIDs (Kurbanov et al. 2003). However, heterosexual contact was considered the main risk factor for infection. From 1987 to 1998, 17,087,645 subjects were examined, and only 51 HIV-positive cases were confirmed (ibid). Of these, 84.3% of cases (43 out of 51 total HIV cases) were not among PWIDs; only 7.8% of the cases (4 out of 51 total HIV cases) until 1998 in Uzbekistan were PWIDs. In other words, the dominant HIV transmission mode between 1987 and 1998 was sexual, but it started rapidly to shift to parenteral transmission after 2000 (ibid). The shift from a (hetero)sexual to an intravenous route of transmission of HIV was observed after 2000, when it accounted for 75% of new cases; in 2001 it accounted for 85% (Kurbanov et al. 2003; UNDP 2008).

The majority of identified HIV cases in the district are among people registered as living in the central town (25), and from three larger regions of the same district (9 from the neighbouring region, 2 cases from a second region and 6 from a third region). Among the newly registered HIV cases, 31% were parenterally transmitted, 27% sexually, and 42% were unknown. According to an AIDS clinic representative, by January 2011, in the district a total of 258 HIV-positive cases were registered. Most were men, but there were 78 women and 26 children (the oldest being 8). Out of 70 PWIDs, 14 were on ART therapy. Today the recent numbers seem to be far below global indicators (Amangaldiyeva et al. 2019). 90-90-90 ART coverage in

Uzbekistan is estimated at 54% in 2020.[5] Only 38% of all people living with HIV were accessing ART in Eastern Europe and Central Asia at the end of 2018, one of the lowest coverage rates in the world (Avert 2019). Although the number of laboratories performing viral load PCR and CD4 counting in Uzbekistan has been gradually increasing recently, they have faced problems obtaining reagents and ART due to their complete dependence on donor funding. Measures are now being taken to facilitate local production of antiretrovirals and HIV testing reagents.

In 2018 the government of Uzbekistan introduced enforced testing for those who spent more than 3 months outside Uzbekistan, as was announced by Dr. K. Abbarov at the Technical Workshop on HIV and Migration for Central Asian Countries and the Russian Federation. According to Dr. Abbarov[6] in 2017, the prevalence of HIV in this category of migrants was 0.15% (in 2016, 2015 and 2014 it was 0.17%, 0.17% and 0.10% respectively). According to the Ministry of Internal Affairs of Russia, as of September 2017, almost six million citizens of five Central Asian states were on the migration register, including 441.853 citizens of Kazakhstan, 640,102 from Kyrgyzstan, 1.586.885 from Tajikistan, 48.173 from Turkmenistan and 3,109,341 from Uzbekistan (a total of 5,826,354 people). The official numbers are not reliable considering the costs and legal constraints for registering migrants in Russia (Turaeva & Urinboyev 2021). Furthermore, Russian migration policies discriminate against people infected with HIV, who face deportation as a result of a positive test, which is another point of concern not only with respect to the reliability of the statistical information on the number of migrants but also the number of returnees.[7] Officially, 5950 migrants have tested positive for HIV infection in Uzbekistan, which is one-sixth of the HIV cases detected in Russia in 2017.[8] All such figures need to be considered in light of the aforementioned barriers and constraints regarding the reliability of statistical information in both Russia and Central Asia.

1.5   The Link Between Drug Abuse and HIV/AIDS

The link between drug abuse and HIV infection is well established by now (Degenhardt et al. 2013; Volkow et al. 2011; NIDA 2021). HIV transmission among PWIDs, remains to be high till today. Harsh drug policies and criminalization laws have targeted PWIDs, with a resultant mass incarceration and prison overcrowding. The literature considering the link between drug abuse and HIV considers largely

---

[5] http://aidsinfo.unaids.org/.

[6] Epidemiologist of the Republican AIDS Centre of the Ministry health care in Uzbekistan.

[7] In accordance with current legislation, the HIV-positive status of a migrant is an obstacle to his entry into Russia and the basis for deportation.

[8] Technical Workshop on HIV and Migration for Central Asian Countries and the Russian Federation, 19–20 February 2018. https://afew.org/wp-content/uploads/2019/11/HIV-REPORT_RUS_FIN_1.pdf.

prison populations, a majority of whom are PWIDs, who suffer from the highest incarceration rates globally (Walmsley 2014).

I will outline the correlation between drug abuse and HIV infection focusing on Central Asia, particularly Uzbekistan. Cheap and easy access to heroin contributed to changes in drug use patterns, from a 'traditional' use of narcotics such as smoking opium and marijuana to intravenous injection of heroin (UNODC 2020). This switch was also supported by drug barons who promoted heroin as a better drug. The shift to a risky administration of drugs can be explained by several factors. One of them is the greater intensity and more rapid onset of euphoria with injection (7–8 s), whereas intramuscular injection produces a slow onset of euphoria (5–8 min), and smoking effects are usually felt within 10–15 min (NIDA 2005). I have been told that around 2000–2001 opium disappeared from Uzbek drug markets. This could be related to policies banning the cultivation of opium poppy in Afghanistan, whereas the decline of opium production led to a shortage of heroin supply in the Uzbek market. Part of this disappearance is said to be related to tighter control by police and the securing of border controls (based on interviews with PWIDs). The disappearance of opium was one of the main reasons that drug users (i.e. opium smokers) switched to heroin. The fact that the heroin supply dropped in times when Western troops entered Afghanistan needs to be newly re-evaluated in the light of 2021 developments in Afghanistan and with the return of the Taliban to power in Afghanistan without Western support.

The preferred drug in the region (Central Asia) was heroin until recently. Over 80% of total registered users are opiate users, with 60–70% injecting opiates in 2008 and 2018 (World Drug Report 2018). In the case of Uzbekistan, of the 70% (in 2008) of drug users who were heroin users, 46% injected drugs. Recent updates on the new patterns of drug consumption among PWIDs in Uzbekistan are nicely visualized in a report by UNODC (2020) based on data gathered from trust points. Trust points are places where drug users are questioned on present drug use habits, which shows the same dangerous trend I myself observed during field research in 2010–2011. The question remains as to why the trend remained the same after the 10 years of my own research presented in 2010–2011 and findings published by UNODC from 2020. This is not the only finding on a particular development of drug abuse which remained unchanged; similar findings have been reported in other fields, such as those described in this book, namely the general approach to public health issues, the general approach to risky behaviour, substance abuse and cultural background, as well as general traditional perceptions about existing problems outlined in this book.

Reports and my research findings support the idea that, due to shortages of drugs and rising prices, PWIDs were shifting to dangerous patterns of drug injection, like injections with Kodatset® (described in Sect. 6.4). Based on data from UNODC (2020:18) collected from trust points, PWID clients indicated that drug users preferred and consumed tablet solutions (53% respondents) for injecting drugs. The same data from trust points (UNODC 2020) indicated an increase in the practice of sharing solutions for injections prepared from a variety of tablet mixtures. There is a high probability that a lack of resources and the right drugs resulted in switching from one type of drug to another. A switch was made from heroin to other alternatives, such as alcohol and pharmacy drugs (UNODC 2020) or injecting a solution made from a confectionery poppy or a substance with the addition of Codeine-containing medicinal products that are self-prepared (these also included gasoline, tea, soda, iodine, sulphur and many others). A recent issue of the World Drug Report 2021 shows the ongoing increase in the demand for synthetic drugs, which accelerated during the early phase of the COVID-19 pandemic as a result of the reduced availability of drugs caused by impediments to the trafficking of cannabis and opiates.

The COVID-19 pandemic also influenced drug patterns and consumption changes among Uzbek PWIDs. According to the data gathered from trust points,[9] due to quarantine measures, supplies of narcotic substances have decreased and accordingly drug prices have increased significantly.

Consequently, increases were seen in the share of clients taking injections of solutions from a variety of tablet mixtures (Bralget and Phenibut instead of Pregabalin) or switching to injecting a solution made from a confectionery poppy. These changes might be explained through problems related to the availability of the right drug (due to restrictions related to COVID-19) or lack of resources and raised drug prices (UNODC 2020).

The switch from smoking to injecting was also observed more in urban than rural settings. The cities and regions with the highest numbers of drug users are reported to be the capital city Tashkent, Kashkadarya, the Khorezm region (which has a high number of registered opiate users), Surkhandarya (bordering Afghanistan and Tajikistan), Jizzak (bordering Tajikistan) and Samarkand (UNODC 2008b). The share of PWIDs who use heroin is 56% in the Namangan region, 22% in the Samarkand region, 8% in the Syrdarya region, 7% in the Khorezm region and the Republic of Karakalpakstan and 1% in the Jizzakh region (UNODC 2020).

It is this shift to injectable drugs that contributed to the rapid rise in HIV cases and produced the concentration of the HIV epidemic in urban areas among the IDU (Injection Drug Users) community. Uzbekistan's youth are recognized as vulnerable to drug abuse and as having limited or no knowledge about HIV/STI infections. Some rapid surveillance to analyse knowledge about HIV/AIDS among young people in Uzbekistan (Sanchez et al. 2006; Boltaev 2017) showed that even knowledge of the danger of infection was not sufficient protection. Many young people reported that they would still engage in risky behaviour (such as non-use of condoms) due to the perception of 'pleasure' or out of a certain kind of 'fatalism'.

I argue that the transition of drug use patterns (from smoking to drug injection) in the region due to ignorance about drugs among the general population, a huge inflow of heroin into Uzbekistan, the restriction of so-called traditional drugs, further tightening of control over drug abuse and sudden disruption of drug inflow has been a crucial development in the outbreak of diseases such as HIV. This, coupled

---

[9] Trust points distribute clean needles and condoms and provide counselling to PWIDs. In 2014 the number of trust points reached 235 (EMCDDA 2014a, b).

with a collapsing healthcare system, poor investments in hygiene and public health, and unprofessional medical personnel, has led to a devastating epidemic in the region. Problems in health care across the region have created situations like that in Kazakhstan and Uzbekistan, where tens of children were infected with HIV in a single hospital (Lillis 2012; Mirovalev 2010; Baigin and Humphries 2010; Vennard 2008). This is only one reported event out of many other dramatic infections that were kept secret in the Central Asian region. Authoritarian regimes enable such secret-keeping and, my local knowledge suggests that many more cases of mass infection were not even investigated because of corrupt judicial systems.

1.6   Gender Aspects of Drug Abuse

Gender is an important aspect of social relations in Central Asia and requires a careful approach and consideration in any analysis. There is a large corpus of scholarly literature considering gender in the region in relation to religion (Harris 2000; Akiner 1997), education (Moghadam 2000), politics and security (Donno and Bruce 2004; Ehteshami 2004; Hoffman 2004; Karatnycky 2002; Lu 2013; Rowley and Nathanael 2009), family relations and marriage (Werner 2004; Tyuryukanova 2011; Turaeva 2011; O'Dea 2016) and human rights (Afkhami and Erika 1997; Baden 1992; Fish 2002) and less related to health- and public health–related themes (Shigakova 2016; Kamiya 2011; Gilbert et al. 2017). Here I would like to focus on the latter, in connection with drug abuse and HIV infection. Infectious diseases which are transferred through sexual intercourse are closely related to issues of family honour (female carriers of family honour are an unimportant aspect of family organization in the Central Asian context), gender relations, generational differences, social status of the relevant family and the economic status of the family. These imply a complete taboo on infections related to sexually transmitted diseases. Substance dependence is another negative category in the social definitions of each individual which are highly gendered. There are important scholarly contributions within the field of gender and drug addiction or gender and infectious diseases depending on political and cultural context of the region considered. The examples (Mohamad 2009; Tahboub et al. 2009) from Muslim-majority countries such as Egypt or UAE show similar patterns of cultural and traditional systems of managing social status and the importance of families within the field of HIV, STIs and drug dependence (Todd et al. 2007; Atilola et al. 2014). This can also be compared to Central Asian countries, where a return to Islam following the collapse of the Soviet Union has been observed (Turaeva 2019; Khalid 2007; McBrien 2009).

Attitudes towards drug users and alcohol abuse are largely gender based. Men can be accepted by their families and their community, whereas women are totally rejected, and their behaviour is largely not accepted. That is to say, men who use drugs also have familial and collective support in the treatment of their drug dependence, whether at home or in hospital, as well as financial support. There is always hope for drug-dependent males will recover. Women, however, are given no chance to correct their behaviour, and once their dependence is discovered, they will be immediately thrown out of their safety nets – family networks, homes and communities. The only chance of survival for such women is to leave home and migrate either to the capital or out of the country. The choice depends on a woman's financial resources and, hence, on her family. From the very beginning, women are financially dependent on their families because of their restricted opportunities in education and career, as well as because of early marriage and the myriad influences of socialization and upbringing.

Exclusion of drug-dependent or alcohol-dependent women from their families and society limits their chances of recovering, let alone being rehabilitated or becoming financially independent. This causes most of these women to turn to sex work. Furthermore, this work is often unsafe due a lack of education on the part of the women and other factors detailed later in this book. Discrimination against female drug users among drug users is no better. Women cannot serve as middlemen or brokers. They are likely to be 'second on the needle' (Harvey et al. 1998), or later within a group, because male PWIDs (including a partner or husband) have dominant control 'over logistics of injection' (Bourgois et al. 2004). This, of course, exposes them to a greater risk of infection than those who inject earlier. Female PWIDs also become an easy target for sexual abuse by policemen. According to Godinho et al. (2005), 10% of all PWIDs in Uzbekistan are female, and 40–50% of them are engaged in sex work in order to subsidize their drug habits. Most of the female drug users I studied were dancers or singers before their drug dependence escalated. Women or work in such fields (singers, dancers and other entertainers) are not traditionally accepted as full family members or potential wives. They tend to come into entertainment work because of problems in their parents' home, and often enough they leave their birth families without marrying. Such women are lucky if they eventually do marry, but otherwise their sexual relations remain outside marriage, and they may offer sex for money. These women are not, however, necessarily prostitutes. Another category of female drug users I got to know during my research were the wives of drug users. Such women may also end up in sex work if (because) their husband is unemployed and there are children in the household.

1.7 Using Ethnographic Methods in Public Health Research in Authoritarian Contexts in Central Asia

The research for this study was designed as a qualitative study of the behavioural patterns and defining social determinants of health behaviour among drug users in Uzbekistan. In the case of Uzbekistan, a qualitative approach indeed led to in-depth insights into the causality of drug use and related infectious diseases, which was otherwise difficult to see because of a lack of reliable (quantitative) statistical information. These approaches help to reveal culturally sensitive categories of HIV knowledge, behaviour in the prevention of HIV infection, attitudes and habits. The research was largely inspired by a Foucauldian approach to studying power and governance through health and biopolitics. The study was designed to collect data not only on individual drug users and other actors but also on institutions (in the broader understanding of the term), behaviour, practices, discourses, legal background, informal and social norms, texts, documents and secondary data. Within the framework of this study there were two clinics, one AIDS centre, 2 NGOs, 2 mahallas (neighbourhoods), and 15 private homes of families of drug users and their neighbours. The number of interviews and persons included in this study was less than the actual number of persons with whom I had contact and whose opinions entered into my general knowledge but are not recorded either in notes or interviews. Only those persons with whom I had systematic contact and whose interviews were recorded entered the sample. The sample of this study is not representative for quantitative research but is rather relevant for qualitative research (Hines 1993). The purposeful sampling (N = 50) with a combination of snowballing techniques was applied based on non-probability principle. The homogeneity of the sample was defined by the limitations of research in a clinical setting with small variations through the use of a snowballing method in the recruitment phase. In what follows I will share the experiences, life stories and other encounters I collected and came across throughout my residence in the region, researching in the same country and learning more about my own country as a public health ethnographer trained in Germany. I came to understand that close engagement with individuals was more helpful in understanding certain complex social relations and other practices than numbers and statistics could tell me about the same issues. I also believe that not everything can be quantified, particularly in the context of secrecy and mistrust in support or intervention programmes in Central Asia.

1.7.1 Limited Ethnography in a Clinical Context

Ethnographic research enables the researcher to enter an individual's or group's daily life in order to find out about the cultural meanings and belief systems connected to certain behaviours, practices, knowledge sharing and other patterns of lifestyle. On the level of a group, it also makes it possible to understand the dynamics and communication within a group which is united through drug dependence. Krefting (1989) used ethnographic methods to study disability, focusing on a particular medical problem to show how and which aspects of daily life were influenced by the problem. I conducted a more limited form of ethnographic study, which I would call clinical ethnography. My ethnography was conducted in lab-like conditions. This has certain advantages in terms of time; it was not necessary to 'hang-out' for long periods of time to gain some form of trust of residents of these clinics and I was able to enter quickly and easily into people's daily routines with the support of the clinic's administration. The main disadvantage is the necessary bias: my informants were attending a narcology clinic. Thus, as an ethnography of a 'medical clinic', it must be understood that this is only a special type of place and space. Similarly, the 'drug users' to whom I had direct and systematic access were those coming to the clinic; the many who have no clinical contacts are necessarily out of focus, although I did engage with the families of the users outside the clinics, as well as close networks of users.

Besides participant observation in the clinic and having meals and participating in other activities discussions together, ethnography in the clinic included participant observation (PO), semi-structured interviews, focus groups and studying documents and photographs. PO as a method was used not only within the clinical setting but also in other places such as events, social gatherings, centres, NGOs and public spaces such as bazars, cafes and parks.

An informal focus group is another method I applied in my study. It is a useful tool for understanding a specific topic from the point of view of the actors and a good tool for cross checking and discussing the same topic. Focus groups offer answers to many questions in a short time period which can also always be asked individually. Observation of interaction is also documented through field notes, and the focus groups are documented through protocols. The disadvantage of focus groups includes the bias or limited environment for individual views on sensitive issues. I was lucky enough to have active participants who led most of the discussions, which accounted for the bias of researchers leading the discussion. The topics for discussion came up during the first phase of the research. I chose the discussion leader after I got to know the group and discuss the issue further with others. The topics to be discussed were decided by the participating PWIDs, who also then led the discussion. The discussion became heated sometimes, and at times it was difficult to intervene. I mainly let group members pursue an open discussion and only entered it when I needed clarification. The focus group discussions were mainly mind-mapped and later recorded in written form.

Mapping cultural settings and events was a useful tool to ensure spatial cultural orientation during the fieldwork considering a very particular kind of navigation of drug users through their specific networks and popular places to meet as well as the designation of each place for different purposes. The places and settings were important to map in order to understand the social networks and the knowledge-sharing methods, means and places popular among drug users.

1.7.2 Target Group

The target group was people with past and present substance abuse, both women and men, above the age of 18. The decision to focus on drug users stemmed from the prevalence of HIV in this group, a fact which had been relied upon to gather statistics before 2010 and which remained relevant to the present day (UNDAF 2021). In 2006, 65.6% of all HIV cases were a result of parenteral infection in Uzbekistan (Wolfe et al. 2008) at the time of the research (2010–2011). The current situation of drug abuse and HIV infection has changed since 2010, the time of the field research for this book; today 72.3% of HIV is transmitted sexually (UNODC

2019). At the time of the field research the target population was chosen as a result of the analysis of statistical information, which implied that injecting drug users made up the majority of those infected with HIV. If I were to do the same research now, I would focus on both PWIDs and their sexual partners, which could be the majority of the population infected by HIV (Avert 2019; LaMonaca et al. 2019) and prison settings, considering harsh drug and other policies and policing targeted at PWIDs in the region. A 2016 study (Altice et al. 2016) estimated that between 28% and 55% of all new HIV infections over the next 15 years in the region will be attributable to heightened HIV transmission risk among currently or previously incarcerated PWIDs. Before arrival in the field, I used existing contacts from previous research and established good contacts with the narcology centres. The recruitment of participants for the actual field research involved several techniques, such as purposeful or targeted sampling, snowball sampling and social networks. Targeted sampling means detecting persons who could be grouped because of a certain feature or behaviour. In the context of this book, it refers to persons who inject drugs intravenously or intramuscularly. Snowball sampling or chain referral (Biemacki and Waldorf 1981) was applied to recruit participants. The following inclusion criteria were used to identify the target group for the research data collection: male and female above 18 years old who had injected drugs in the 6 months preceding the time of the interview. Groups not included in the sampling were drug users younger than 18 years old (during my research stays in both narcology centres there were no patients younger than 18), people who abused alcohol but no other drugs and people who did not use drugs by injection. A financial incentive was offered in return for interviews to PWIDs recruited outside of clinical settings. Inside the clinics, invitations to coffee with sweets were appreciated by PWIDs. Outside of clinical settings, I relied on a connection with an influential woman trusted and respected by my informants. After her personal referral I was automatically treated as a trusted person.[10]

The 50 research participants who were recruited for in-depth interviews came from different cities. Twenty-five (21 male, 4 female) were recruited from a narcology centre in the capital city.[11] Another 17 PWIDs (13 male, 4 female) were recruited from a narcology centre in another district (a small city with a population of 1.5 million) (The Senate of the Oliy Majlis of the Republic of Uzbekistan 2018). These 42 interviews were conducted within the two clinics. The remaining eight participants were recruited from outside of narcology centres with the help of an AIDS clinic referral, NEP referral, and other private connections.

---

[10] Being recommended by a highly respected person is a very common and necessary strategy in Uzbekistan. It is a very common strategy used by all people to gain access to places or people, achieve success in one's career, gain some sort of financial benefit, and so forth; it is even sometimes enough to say that you are related to some powerful person while being detained by the militia or police to avoid paying a bribe.

[11] Tashkent had a population of 2,545,159 million in 2021 (World Population Review website, http://worldpopulationreview.com/countries/uzbekistan-population/).

1.7.3 Fieldwork and Field Sites

The field research was conducted in two phases. The first phase of the field research ran from September 2010 to February 2011. It was during this time that the central 50 interviews were recorded.

The second phase of field work for updating the data was conducted from October 2011 to the end of November 2011. During this time, I conducted additional interviews and had conversations with health professionals, authorities in the field of health management and public health centres, as well as the other experts mentioned previously. Until 2015, contacts with main informants were kept active via online applications, messengers, phone and indirect contact. During the second phase of field research, I also conducted archival research on the history of drug consumption. It included sources from the Tashkent national library and Urgench regional libraries. It was necessary to do this research in situ because most of the relevant Soviet literature is available only in hard copy. Prior to beginning even the first stage of fieldwork, I amassed data which showed basic local conceptions and trends in HIV/AIDS in the target group. This was done with preliminary interviews with 'stakeholders', *mahhalla* (neighbourhood) members and local community members. The stakeholders, as I defined them, included health professionals from the ministry of health, narcologists, directors of narcology centres, AIDS clinic representatives and trust point representatives (September 2010).

Research was conducted in two districts of Uzbekistan. The two districts are not comparable in terms of size or infrastructure. Rather, they represent two very different social and cultural contexts. The statistical information used for the selection of the field sites, however, considered the registered number of drug users and concentration of HIV infection. The capital was one of the field sites. The other was in a district traditionally known for opium consumption: it is an integral part of party culture (culturally close to Turkmenistan), and opium is a traditional medicine used in the treatment of headaches, diarrhoea (even given to children) and other diseases. One of the selected regions in this district is a close border region and contributes to traffic routes and drug consumption patterns. The region itself is notorious for the high prevalence of drug abuse and spread of HIV (Kerimi and Ladygina 1991). A security officer told me in conversation that the region is a focus of the country's drug prevention agency. As for the capital, it is located along a drug-trafficking route that comes from Afghanistan – the world's biggest drug supplier (UNODC 2011) – and it is the centre for most of the HIV/AIDS preventive programmes in the country. After the rise of the Taliban to power, it remains to be seen how drug trafficking will change and what those changes will bring to the region in terms of drug abuse and other insecurities related to the refugee crisis.

1.7.4   Ethical Issues

European ethical rules for collecting data were considered when designing this research. Informed oral consent was collected from each informant with whom I had an interview, informal conversation or other contact. Agreements were also made regarding the ways the data should be treated in the future. It was agreed that I would not share the raw data I collected, that only the results would be published, and that the informants would be anonymized. The printed interview transcripts submitted to the university contain no details which could identify or help to locate the informants. All names and other personal identifiers of informants included in this book have been changed to protect their privacy and confidentiality. Reciprocity rules have also been kept to the degree acceptable by both me and my informants. Research participants were remunerated by both non-monetary and monetary compensation. I also served as an information source on various health issues, including HIV, TB, HCV and STIs. I also provided them with informational booklets obtained from AIDS clinics and TB centres. Non-monetary incentives included invitations for dinner, drinks in cafes and other small gifts.

For research participants recruited outside of the narcology centres, confidentiality and security were expressly guaranteed. The meeting point was chosen by the participants themselves in neutral areas where they felt secure. Participants' identity (PWIDs, CSWs) was kept anonymous. Participants were free to choose a nickname for themselves in the study, meaning that I never knew their real names.

1.7.5   Data Analysis

The study used a phenomenological approach to analyse the collected data. Part of the intent was to explain the lived experience of drug dependence and what it is like to be a drug user in Uzbekistan. This approach considers all forms of experience of drug users themselves as well as their own reflections about their lives. Even before data analysis, this approach presumes a qualitative stance. It imagines that a researcher can reconstruct the daily lives and practices under study. The approach taken by Dyck and Forwell (1997) was largely helpful throughout the study and its analysis. The data were managed using memo notes during the transcription as well as reading the transcripts. Textual analysis (content analysis) was applied to analyse the qualitative data. Analysis was ongoing throughout the data collection and transcription phases of the study. Throughout the process of interview transcription, memos were recorded in the margins, reflecting the identification of emerging themes. Memo writing (field notes) is a strategy utilized in qualitative analysis to aid in the conceptual development of raw data into abstracted explanations by clarifying thinking, articulating assumptions, and retaining ideas (Birks et al. 2008; Glaser 1978). During the transcription phase, memos were used to identify a priori themes corresponding to patterns of drug use, behavioural patterns, identity, social factors or other social and institutional settings. The themes were established based on the prior knowledge of the researcher (Ryan and Bernard 2003). For this study, theoretical explanations of behavioural patterns, social determinants of health, the institutional set-up of treatment and punitive regimes were the leading themes.

All texts were reviewed for patterns occurring around the aforementioned themes. In this process of textual analysis, categories were identified and subdivided into further subcategories and systematized according to the frequency of occurrence, emphasis made by practices and explanations of my informants. The analytical and reflective work was conducted over the whole period of research during and after fieldwork. Furthermore, the data were then interpreted based on the context of the responses and the strength of the comments in terms of frequency, emotion and specificity (Krueger 1988; Glaser 1965). Analytic coding was used during the process of noting and memo writing to compare themes (by linking, summarizing, and analysing the data to define concepts and categories) (Richards and Morse 2007).

Other data (secondary material, notes, video, photo and other visual data, SMS texts and other files shared within smartphone applications) entered into the general knowledge base and information about relevant issues. These sources contained information on social status, gender roles, social determinants of health, risky behaviour, social control systems, principles of administration of health and punitive regimes. Tones, gestures, the ways in which social lives were organized, and social relations were maintained and entered the reflections and interpretations of the more formally gathered data.

1.7.6 Interviews

In-depth interviews are also known as *face-to-face* interviews, which explore particular topics through guided conversations. The in-depth interviews were '*open*' and '*non-directive*' (Rhodes and Coomber 2010). Other forms of interviewing used included *telephone interviews*, communication through mobile applications such as Telegram and IMO. Contact with key informants was maintained for several years after the fieldwork, which was useful for clarifying certain questions that arose in the analysis of the data, as well as for updating the data about recent trends in drug abuse. The questionnaire for the interviews was developed to include questions on social aspects of the daily lives of drug users, educational background, family background, employment, social networks, information on drugs and drug use patterns, social status, identity, daily concerns and life events.

The in-depth interviews were conducted with representatives of local NGOs, AIDS clinics, narcologists, local leaders, community members, PWIDs' wives and ex-police officers. The study included 2 narcology clinics, 1 AIDS clinic, 2 NGOs, 2 *mahallas*, 4 police officers and 15 families (7 in Tashkent, 8 in Urgench). Sixteen interviews included seven narcologists, one person from the AIDS clinic, two men on a *mahallas* committee and four police officers. Expert interviews were conducted with the medical personnel of the narcology clinics, private doctors, and nurses who privately showed up to carry out cleaning infusions for drug users treated at home. Additional expert interviews with NGO workers, trust point[12] representatives, neighbourhood (*mahalla*) committees,[13] police officers and government officials were also conducted. In total, I recorded and transcribed 50 interviews with drug users. This does not include informal chats, conversations or telephone interactions. An additional 16 interviews were not audio-recorded, though I took handwritten notes. Most of these were with state officials who refused an audio-recording but did not mind my taking notes. After I contextualized the data I collected during my fieldwork and explained the positioning of myself as a native female researcher, it was easier to imagine what data were going to be analysed later. Before I outline the contents of the same data, I will also contextualize the regional and historical background. The next chapter is not simply a history of drug abuse, which will not be very helpful for understanding the current epidemiological situation in a context such as Central Asia; rather, following a particular approach to making connections such as that offered by Foucault, I will try to outline the genealogy of drug abuse and HIV infection in Central Asia.

References

Afkhami M, Erika F, editors. Muslim women and the politics of participation. New York: Syracuse University Press; 1997.

Akiner S. Between tradition and modernity: the dilemma facing contemporary Central Asian women. In: Buckley M, editor. Post-Soviet women: from the Baltic to Central Asia. Cambridge: Cambridge University Press; 1997. p. 261–304.

Alexandrova L. Human rights of people living with HIV in Tajikistan. The Foreign Policy Centre; 2021. https://fpc.org.uk/human-rights-of-people-living-with-hiv-in-tajikistan/.

Altice FL, Azbel L, Stone J, Brooks-Pollock E, Smyrnov P, Dvoriak S, Taxman FS, El-Bassel, Nabila M, Natasha K, Booth R, Stöver H, Dolan K, Vickerman P. The perfect storm: Incarceration and the high-risk environment perpetuating transmission of HIV, hepatitis C virus, and tuberculosis in Eastern Europe and Central Asia. Lancet. 2016;388(10050):1228–48.

Amangaldiyeva A, Davlidova S, Baiserkin B, et al. Implementation of antiretroviral therapy (ART) in former Soviet Union countries. AIDS Res Ther. 2019;16(35). https://doi.org/10.1186/s12981-019-0251-1.

Ancker S, Rechel B. Policy responses to HIV/AIDS in Central Asia. Glob Public Health. 2015;10(7):817–33. https://doi.org/10.1080/17441692.2015.1043313.

Antonov O, Edward L. Responses to COVID-19 and the strengthening of authoritarian governance in Central Asia. In: Laruelle M, editor. COVID-19 pandemic and Central Asia crisis management, economic impact, and social transformations. Central Asia Program, The George Washington University, Washington, D.C; 2021. p. 51–61.

Archin NM, Margolis DM. Emerging strategies to deplete the HIV reservoir. Curr Opin Infect Dis. 2014;27(1):29–35. https://doi.org/10.1097/QCO.0000000000000026.

---

[12] Trust Points distribute clean needles and condoms and provide counselling to PWIDs.

[13] These committees are very active in community life. They tend to be aware of problems in each household of the community and try to help financially, with recommendations and connections.

Atilola O, Stevanovic D, Balhara YP, Avicenna M, Kandemir H, Knez R, Petrov P, Franic T, Vostanis P. Role of personal and family factors in alcohol and substance use among adolescents: an international study with focus on developing countries. J Psychiatr Ment Health Nurs. 2014;21:609–17.

Avert. HIV and AIDS in Eastern Europe & Central Asia overview. 2019. https://www.avert.org/hiv-and-aids-eastern-europe-central-asia-overview#footnote37_gwyjtsq.

Baden S. The position of women in Islamic countries: possibilities, constraints and strategies for change. Report prepared for the Special Programme WID, Netherlands Ministry of Foreign Affairs (DGIS). Brighton: Institute of Development Studies; 1992.

Baigin S, Humphries C. 147 children infected with HIV in Uzbekistan—report. London: Reuters; 2010. http://www.alertnet.org/thenews/newsdesk/LDE62L1ME.htm. Accessed 11 May 2010.

Baillargeon J, Pulvino JS, Leonardson JE, Linthicum LC, Williams B, Penn J, et al. The changing epidemiology of HIV in the criminal justice system. Int J STD AIDS. 2017;28(13):1335–40.

Barton KM, Burch BD, Soriano-Sarabia N, Margolis DM. Prospects for treatment of latent HIV. Clin Pharmacol Ther. 2013;93(1):46–56. https://doi.org/10.1038/clpt.2012.202.

Biemacki P, Waldorf D. Snowball sampling: problems and techniques in chain-referral sampling. Sociol Methods Res. 1981;10:141–63.

Birks M, Chapman Y, Francis K. Memoing in qualitative research: probing data and processes. J Res Nurs. 2008;13:68–75.

Boltaev MP. Gender aspects of HIV infection in Eastern Europe and Central Asia. 2017. http://congress-ph.ru/common/htdocs/upload/fm/vich/17/prez/5-A3-4.pdf.

Bourgois P, Prince B, Moss A. The everyday violence of hepatitis C among young women who inject drugs in San Francisco. Hum Organ. 2004;63:253–64.

Brill Olcott M, Aslund A, Garnett SW. Getting it wrong: regional cooperation and the commonwealth of independent states. Washington, DC: Carnegie Endowment for Int'l Peace; 2000.

Burkle FM. Declining public health protections within autocratic regimes: impact on global public health security, infectious disease outbreaks, epidemics, and pandemics. Prehosp Disaster Med. 2020;00(00):1–10.

Campbell Nancy D. Discovering addiction: the science and politics of substance abuse research. Ann Arbor: University of Michigan Press; 2007.

CARICC. Information Bulletin, No. 213. Sept 2020.

Degenhardt L, Whiteford HA, Ferrari AJ, et al. Global burden of disease attributable to illicit drug use and dependence: findings from the Global Burden of Disease Study 2010. Lancet Lond Engl. 2013;382(9904):1564–1574. https://doi.org/10.1016/S0140-6736(13)61530-5.

Degenhardt L, Peacock A, Colledge S, Leung J, Grebely J, Vickerman P, et al. Global prevalence of injecting drug use and sociodemographic characteristics and prevalence of HIV, HBV, and HCV in people who inject drugs: a multistage systematic re-view. Lancet Glob Health. 2017. https://doi.org/10.1016/S2214-109X(17)30375-3.

Dehne KL, Khodakevich L, Hamers FF, Schwartländer B. The HIV/AIDS epidemic in Eastern Europe: recent patterns and trends and their implications for policymaking. AIDS. 1999;13(7):741–9.

DeHovitz J, Uuskula A, El-Bassel N. The HIV epidemic in Eastern Europe and Central Asia. Curr HIV/AIDS Rep. 2014;11:168–76.

Donno D, Bruce R. Islam, authoritarianism and empowerment: what are the linkages? World Polit. 2004;56(4):582–607.

Donoghoe MC, Lazarus JV, Matic S. HIV/AIDS in the transitional countries of Eastern Europe and Central Asia. Clin Med. 2005;2005(5):487–90.

Dyck I, Forwell S. Cultural issues in fieldwork: first year occupational therapy student experiences. Can J Occup Ther. 1997;62:185–96.

Ehteshami A. Islam, Muslim polities and democracy. Democratization. 2004;11(4):90–110.

Fish MS. Islam and authoritarianism. World Polit. 2002;55(1):4–37. https://doi.org/10.1353/wp.2003.

Foucault M. The ethics of the concern for self as a practice of freedom. In: Foucault M, Rabinow PD, editors. Essential works of Foucault 1954–1984, vol. 1: ethics: subjectivity and truth. New York, Penguin Books; 1997. p. 281–302.

Gilbert L, Jiwatram-Negron T, Nikitin D, Rychkova O, McCrimmon T, Ermolaeva I, Hunt T. Feasibility and preliminary effects of a screening, brief intervention and referral to treatment model to address gender-based violence among women who use drugs in Kyrgyzstan: Project WINGS (Women Initiating New Goals of Safety). Drug Alcohol Rev. 2017;36(1):125–33. https://doi.org/10.1111/dar.12437.

Glaser BG. The constant comparative method of qualitative analysis. Soc Probl. 1965;12(4):436–45. https://doi.org/10.1525/sp.1965.12.4.03a00070.

Glaser BG. Theoretical sensitivity: advances in the methodology of grounded theory. Mill Valley: Sociology Press; 1978.

Godinho J, Renton A, Vinogradov V, Novotny T, Rivers MJ, Gotsadze G, Bravo M. Reversing the tide: priorities for HIV/AIDS prevention in Central Asia. World Bank Working Paper No. 54. Washington, DC: World Bank. © World Bank; 2005. https://openknowledge.worldbank.org/handle/10986/7354 License: CC BY 3.0 IGO.

Harris C. The changing identity of women in Tajikistan in the post-Soviet period. In: Acar F, Gunes-Ayata A, editors. Gender and identity construction: women in Central Asia, the Caucasus, and Turkey. Boston: Leiden; 2000. p. 205–28.

Harvey E, Strathdee SA, Patrick DM, Ofner M, Archibald CP, Eades G, O'Shaughnessy MV. A qualitative investigation into an HIV outbreak among injection drug users in Vancouver, British Columbia. AIDS Care. 1998;10:313–21.

Hines AM. Linking qualitative and quantitative methods in cross-cultural survey research: techniques from cognitive science. Am J Community Psychol. 1993;21:729–46.

Hoffman SR. Islam and democracy: micro-level indications of compatibility. Comp Pol Stud. 2004;37(6):652–76.

Hohlov I. *Proizvodstvo opiynuh narkotikov (geroina) v Afganistane: infrastruktura narkobiznessa* (Production of drugs of opium (heroin) in Afganistan: infrastructure of narcobusiness). Institute of World Economy and International Relations. Russian Academy of Science; 2006. http://www.nationalsecurity.ru/library/00021/index.htm.

IHRD. Harm reduction developments 2008. New York: International Harm Reduction Development Program of the Open Society Institute; 2008.

IISS. Central Asia's narcotic industry. Strategic Comments. 1997;3:5:1–2.

International Narcotics Control Board. Vienna International Centre. INCB; 2020.

Kamiya Y. Women's autonomy and reproductive health care utilisation: empirical evidence from Tajikistan. Health Policy. 2011;102(2–3):304–13. https://doi.org/10.1016/j.healthpol.2011.04.001.

Karatnycky A. Muslim countries and the democracy gap. J Democr. 2002;13(1):99–112.

Kerimi NB, Ladygina LS. Dinamika Zabolevaemosti I Boleznennosti Opiinoi Narkomaniei v Turkmenistane v 1959–1988gg. (Dynamics of morbidity and soreness of opium drug addiction in Turkmenistan in 1959–1988th). Voprosy narkologii. 1991;2:25–8.

Khalid A. Islam after communism: religion and politics in Central Asia. Islam after communism: religion and politics in Central Asia. Berkeley: University of California Press; 2007. p. 260.

Krefting L. Disability ethnography: a methodological approach for occupational therapy research. Can J Occup Ther. 1989;56:61–6.

Krueger RA. Focus groups: a practical guide for applied research. Thousand Oaks: Sage; 1988.

Kukeyeva F, Shkapyak O. Central Asia' s transition to democracy. Procedia Soc Behav Sci. 2013;81:79–83.

Kupatadze A. Organized crime, political transitions and state formation in post-Soviet Eurasia. London: Palgrave Macmillan UK; 2012.

Kupatadze A. Kyrgyzstan – a virtual narco-state? Int J Drug Policy. 2014;25(6):1178–85. https://doi.org/10.1016/j.drugpo.2014.01.012.

Kurbanov F, Kondo M, Tanaka Y, Zalalieva M, Glasova G, Shimat T, Jounai N, Yuldasheva N, Ruzibakiev R, Mizokami M, Imai M. Human immunodeficiency virus in Uzbekistan: epidemiological and genetic analyses. AIDS Res Hum Retrovir. 2003;19:731–8.

LaMonaca K, Dumchev KS, Azbel L, Morozova O, Altice FL. HIV, drug injection, and harm reduction trends in Eastern Europe and Central Asia: implications for international and domestic policy. Curr Psychiatry Rep. 2019;21:47.

Leshner AI. Addiction is a brain disease, and it matters. Science. 1997;278(5335):45.

Lillis J. Kazakhstan: Shymkent's HIV scandal, six years later. https://eurasianet.org/kazakhstan-shymkents-hiv-scandal-six-years-later. 2012. Accessed in Mar 2015.

Lu SFDP. Women's electoral participation in Muslim majority and Non-Mulsim majority countries. J Int Women's Stud. 2013;14(3):137–47.

Lundgren JD, Raben D, Eramova I, Ilyenkova V. HIV/AIDS treatment and care in Belarus evaluation report January 2014. WHO Regional Office for Europe; 2014. https://www.euro.who.int/__data/assets/pdf_file/0008/246617/ENG-Belarus_report_Final-for-web-with-cover.pdf.

Mathers BM, Degenhardt L, Phillips BT, Wiessing L, Hickman M, Strathdee SA, Wodak A, Panda S, Tyndall M, Toufik A, Mattick RP. Global epidemiology of injecting drug use and HIV among people who inject drugs: a systematic review. Lancet. 2008;372:1733–45.

Mathers BM, Degenhardt L, Ali H, Wiessing L, Hickman M, Mattick RP, et al. HIV prevention, treatment and care services for people who inject drugs a systematic review of global, regional and national coverage. Lancet. 2010;375(9719):1014–28.

McBrien J. Mukadas's struggle: veils and modernity in Kyrgyzstan. J R Anthropol Inst. 2009;15:127–44.

McKee M, Rechel B, Richardson E, editors. Trends in health systems in the former Soviet countries. The European Observatory on Health Systems; 2014. https://www.euro.who.int/__data/assets/pdf_file/0019/261271/Trends-in-health-systems-in-the-former-Soviet-countries.pdf.

Michels I, Keizer B, Trautmann F, Stoever H, Robelló E. Improvement of treatment of drug use disorders in Central Asia the contribution of the EU Central Asia Drug Action Programme (CADAP). J Addict Med Ther. 2017;5(1):1025.

Michels I, Aizberg O, Boltaev A, Stoever H. Opioid agonist treatment for opioid use disorder patients in Central Asia. Heroin Addict Relat Clin Probl. 2021;23(1):33–46.

Mirovalev M. Film: 147 toddlers infected in Uzbek HIV outbreak. 2010. https://www.seattletimes.com/seattle-news/health/film-147-toddlers-infected-in-uzbek-hiv-outbreak/. Accessed 7 Oct 2010.

Moghadam V. Gender and economic reforms: a framework for analysis and evidence from Central Asia, the Caucasus, and Turkey. In: Acar F, Gunes-Ayata A, editors. Gender and identity construction: women in Central Asia, the Caucasus, and Turkey. Boston: Brill; 2000.

Mohamad MS. Daily hassles, coping strategies, and substance use among Egyptian manufacturing workers. J Muslim Ment Health. 2009;4(1):17–29. https://doi.org/10.1080/15564900902774097.

Mounier S, McKee M, Atun R, Coker R. HIV/AIDS in Central Asia. In: Twigg JL, editor. HIV/AIDS in Russia and Eurasia, vol. 2. New York: Palgrave Macmillan; 2006.

NIDA. Heroin abuse and addiction. Bethesda: National Institute on Drug Abuse; 2005.

NIDA. Part 1: the connection between substance use disorders and mental illness. 2021, April 13. https://www.drugabuse.gov/publications/research-reports/common-comorbidities-substance-use-disorders/part-1-connection-between-substance-use-disorders-mental-illness. Accessed 6 Sept 2021.

O'Dea C. The growth and influence of Islam in the nations of Asia and Central Asia: Tajikistan. Philadelphia: Mason Crest Publishers; 2016.

Peyrouse S. The Health of the Nation—the Wealth of the Homeland! Turkmenistan's Potemkin Healthcare System. PONARS Eurasia Policy Memo No. 574. 2019. https://www.ponarseurasia.org/wp-content/uploads/attachments/Pepm574_Peyrouse_Feb2019.pdf.

Platt L, French CE, McGowan CR, Sabin K, Gower E, Trickey A, et al. Prevalence and burden of HBV co-infection among people living with HIV: a global systematic review and meta-analysis. J Viral Hepat. 2020;27(3):294–315.

Rechel B, et al. Lessons from two decades of health reform in Central Asia. Health Policy Plan. 2012a;27(4):281–7.

Rechel B, Ahmedov M, Akkazieva B, Katsaga A, Khodjamurodov G, McKee M. Lessons from two decades of health reform in Central Asia. Health Policy Plan. 2012b;7(4):1–7.

Rechel B, et al. Health and health systems in the commonwealth of independent states. Lancet. 2013;381(9872):1145–55.

Rhodes T, Coomber R. Qualitative methods and theory in addictions research. In: Miller PG, Strang J, Miller PM, editors. Addiction research methods. Oxford: Blackwell Publishing Ltd; 2010.

Rhodes T, Simic M. Transition and the HIV risk environment. BMJ. 2005;331:220–3.

Richards L, Morse JM. Readme first for a user's guide to qualitative methods. Thousand Oaks: Sage Publications; 2007.

Rowley CK, Nathanael S. Islam's democracy paradox: Muslims claim to like democracy, So Why Do They Have So Little? Public Choice. 2009;139:273–99.

Ryan GW, Bernard H. Techniques to identify themes. Field Methods. 2003;15(1):85–109. https://doi.org/10.1177/1525822X02239569.

Sanchez JL, Todd CS, Earhart KC, Botros BA, Khakimov MM, Giyasova GM, Bautista CT, Carr JK. High HIV prevalence and risk factors among injection drug users in Tashkent, Uzbekistan, 2003–2004. Drug Alcohol Depend. 2006;82(Suppl 1):15–S22.

Shigakova FA. Group psychotherapy in rehabilitation of female opium addicts in Uzbekistan. Int J Group Psychother. 2016;66(1):120–31. https://doi.org/10.1080/00207284.2015.1089692.

Smolak A, Nabila El-Bassel N, Malin A, Terlikbayeva A, Samatova S. Sex workers, condoms, and mobility among men in Uzbekistan: implications for HIV transmission. Int J STD AIDS. 2016;27(4):268–72.

Stoever H. Opioid substitution treatment (OST) for prisoners: practices, problems and perspectives [Substitutionsbehandlung mit Opioiden für Strafgefangene: Praxis, Probleme und Zukunftsperspektiven]. Akzeptanzorientierte Drogenarbeit/Acceptance-Oriented Drug Work. 2010;7:20–32.

Stoever H, Azbel L, Stone J, Brooks-Pollock E, Smyrnov P, Dvoriak S, Taxman F, El-Bassel N, Martin N, Booth R, Dolan K, Vickerman P. The perfect storm: incarceration and the high-risk environment perpetuating transmission of HIV, hepatitis C virus, and tuberculosis in Eastern Europe and Central Asia. The Lancet. 2016;388. https://doi.org/10.1016/S0140-6736(16)30856-X.

Stoever H, Schäffer D, Knorr B, Dettmer K. Hepatitis C und Drogengebrauch: Grundlagen, Therapie, Prävention, Betreuung, Recht. Ein Handbuch; 2019.

Stoever H, Moazen B, Dolan K, Albrecht J, Neuhann F. Prisoners should not be left behind in HCV research and policies. Harm Reduct J. 2020;17. https://doi.org/10.1186/s12954-020-00379-y.

Stone K, Shirley-Beavan S. Global state of harm reduction 2018. London: Harm Reduction International; 2018.

Storti C, De Grauwe P. Globalization and the price decline of illicit drugs. Int J Drug Policy. 2009;20(1):48–61. https://doi.org/10.1016/j.drugpo.2007.11.016.

Tahboub-Schulte S, Ali AY, Khafaji T. Treating substance dependency in the UAE: a case study. J Muslim Ment Health. 2009;4(1):67–75. https://doi.org/10.1080/15564900902787578.

The European Monitoring Centre for Drugs and Drug Addiction. Tajikistan country overview 2014. EMCDDA, 2014a. Available in: https://www.emcdda.europa.eu/publications/country-overviews/tj_en.

The European Monitoring Centre for Drugs and Drug Addiction. Overview of the drug situation in Uzbekistan (2014). EMCDDA, 2014b. Available in: https://www.emcdda.europa.eu/publications/country-overviews/uzbekistan-2014.

The Senate of the Oliy Majlis of the Republic of Uzbekistan. Brief political and socio-economic background of the regions of Uzbekistan and the Republic of Karakalpakstan. 2018. http://

senat.uz/en/senate-slrp/brief-political-and-socio-economic-backgrounds.html. Accessed 20 Mar 2018.

Todd CS, Nassiramanesh B, Stanekzai MR, et al. Emerging HIV epidemics in Muslim countries: assessment of different cultural responses to harm reduction and implications for HIV control. Curr HIV/AIDS Rep. 2007;4:151–7. https://doi.org/10.1007/s11904-007-0022-9.

Turaeva M. Feminization of trade in post-Soviet Central Asia. In: Kahlert H, Schäfer S, editors. Engendering transformation. Post-socialist experiences on work, politics and culture. Special issue of GENDER. Zeitschrift für Geschlecht, Kultur und Gesellschaft Opladen: Budrich Verlag; 2011. p. 26–39.

Turaeva R. Imagined mosque communities in Russia: Central Asian migrants in Moscow. Asian Ethn. 2019;20(2):131–47. https://doi.org/10.1080/14631369.2018.152552.

Turaeva M, Turaeva R. *Uchyot* and Foucault: drug users and migration in Uzbekistan. Cent Asian Aff. 2021;8:83–98.

Turaeva R & Urinboyev R. (Eds). Labour, Mobility and Informal Practices in Russia, Central Asia and Eastern Europe: Power, Institutions and Mobile Actors in Transnational Space - BASEES / Routledge Series on Russian and East European Studies. Routledge. 2021. https://doi.org/10.4324/9781003176763.

Tyuryukanova YV, editor. *Zhenshhiny-migranty iz stran SNG v Rossii* [Female migrants from the CIS States in Russia]. Moscow: MAX Press; 2011.

UNAIDS. UNAIDS data 2019. Geneva, Switzerland; 2019a. https://www.unaids.org/sites/default/files/media_asset/2019-UNAIDS-data_en.pdf.

UNAIDS (2016). Global AIDS Update 2016. Joint United Nations Programme on HIV/AIDS (UNAIDS). UNAIDS, 2016 Country Profile: Kazakhstan. Available at http://www.unaids.org/.

UNAIDS. Global HIV & AIDS statistics-2019 Fact Sheet. HIV/AIDS JUNPo. The Gap Report. Geneva: UNAIDS; 2019b. p. 2014–2015.

UNAIDS. United Nations Development Assistance Framework (UNDAF), 2016–2020. Uzbekistan United Nations Country Report 2019c.

UNAIDS Data 2020. Key HIV indicators – AIDS info: UZBEKISTAN. http://aidsinfo.unaids.org/. UNAIDS Data 2018. https://www.unaids.org/en/resources/documents/2018/unaids-data-2018.

UNDAF. Uzbekistan United Nations Country results report 2019 United Nations Development Assistance Framework (UNDAF) 2016–2020. 2021. https://unsdg.un.org/sites/default/files/2021-02/PDF.pdf.

UNDP Report. Qualitative analysis for the assessment of social implications of HIV and identification of advocacy priorities in Uzbekistan. United Nations Development Programme (UNDP); 2008.

United Nations Development Assistance Framework. Uzbekistan United Nations Country results report 2019. UNDAF; 2019.

United Nations Office on Drugs and Crime. Afghan opiate trafficking along the northern route. Vienna: United Nations Office on Drugs and Crime; 2018.

United Nations Office on Drugs and Crime. Annual report 2019 together making the region safer from drugs, crime and terrorism. UNODC Regional Office for Central Asia; 2019.

United Nations publication, Sales No. E.18.XI.9. 2018. https://www.unodc.org/wdr2018/pre-launch/WDR18_Booklet_1_EXSUM.pdf.

UNODC, 2009. Addiction, Crime and insurgency: The transnational threat of Afghan opium. United Nations Office on Drugs and Crime.

UNODC. World drug report 2010. United Nations Publication, Sales No. E.10.XI.13; 2010.

UNODC Report. Compendium drug related statistics. United Nations Office on Drugs and Crime Regional Office for Central Asia; 2008a.

UNODC Report. Illicit drug trends in Central Asia. United Nations Office on Drugs and Crime Regional Office for Central Asia; 2008b.

UNODC Report. The global Afghan opium trade: a threat assessment. United Nations Office on Drugs and Crime; 2011.

UNODC Report. Brief overview of COVID-19 impact on drug use situation as well as on the operations of the drug treatment services and harm reduction programmes in Central Asia. 2020. https://www.unodc.org/documents/centralasia/2020/August/3.08/COVID-19_impact_on_drug_use_in_Central_Asia_en.pdf.

Valverde M. Diseases of the will: alcohol and the dilemmas of freedom. Cambridge: Cambridge University Press; 1998.

Vennard M. Uzbek children in "HIV outbreak". BBC News. 2008. http://news.bbc.co.uk/go/pr/fr/-/2/hi/asia-pacific/7722735.stm. Accessed Jan 2010.

Volkow ND, Baler RD, Normand JL. The unrealized potential of addiction science in curbing the HIV epidemic. Curr HIV Res. 2011;9(6):393–5.

Vranken MJM, Mantel-Teeuwisse AK, Junger S, Radbruch L, Scholten W, Lisman JA, et al. Barriers to access to opioid medicines for patients with opioid dependence: a review of legislation and regulations in eleven central and eastern European countries. Addiction. 2017;112(6):1069–76. https://doi.org/10.1111/add.13755.

Vrecko S. Folk neurology and the remaking of identity. Mol Interv. 2006;6(6):300–3.

Walmsley R. World prison population list. 10th ed. London: University of Essex; 2014.

Werner C. Feminizing the new silk road: women traders in rural Kazakhstan. In: Kuehnast K, Nechemias C, editors. Post-Soviet women encountering transition: nation building, economic survival, and civic activism. Baltimore: Johns Hopkins University Press; 2004.

Wolfe D, Elovich R, Boltaev A, Pulatov D. Public health aspects of HIV/AIDS in low- and middle-income countries epidemiology, prevention and care. In: Celantano DD, Beyrer C, editors. Public health aspects of HIV/AIDS in low- and middle-income countries: epidemiology, prevention and care. New York: Springer; 2008. p. 557–81.

World Drug Report. United Nations publication, Sales No. E.21.XI.8. 2021.

World Drug Report (2018) United Nations Report 2018. World Drug Report 2018 Pre-briefing to the Member States. Viena.

World Health Organisation. Global HIV, Hepatitis and STIs Programmes. WHO; 2021.

Zabransky T, Mravcik V, editors. The 2019 regional report on the drug situation in Central Asia [Reguonalnuy obzor o narkosituatsii v Sentralnoy Azii 2019]. Bishkek/Prague: CADAP 6/ResAd; 2019.

Zabransky T, Talu A, Jasaitis E, Mravcik V. Post-Soviet Central Asia: a summary of the drug situation. Int J Drug Policy. 2014;25(6):1186–94. https://doi.org/10.1016/j.drugpo.2014.05.004. Epub 2014 May 21.

Zhao F, Clemens B, Wilson D, editors. Tackling the world's fastest-growing HIV epidemic: more efficient HIV responses in Eastern Europe and Central Asia. Human development perspectives. Washington, DC: World Bank; 2020. https://doi.org/10.1596/978-1-4648-1523-2. License: Creative Commons Attribution CC BY 3.0 IGO.

Chapter 2
Genealogy of Drug Abuse and HIV Infection in Central Asia

This chapter will trace the genealogies of drug abuse and HIV infection in Central Asia. I use the concept of genealogy following the definitions of Foucault. Foucault advanced Nietzsche's approach, namely that genealogy as the method furthered in his *Archeology of Knowledge* and *Genealogy, Nietzsche and History*. According to Foucauldian genealogy, unlike history or archeology, where the latter are the processes of tracing objects and knowledge from existing textual facts and selected sources, genealogy as a method includes a broader historical enquiry of relevant objects, discourses, images and many more things which provide a better understanding of the phenomenon in question. When defining genealogy, Foucault observed: 'Genealogy does not oppose itself to history as the lofty and profound gaze of the philosopher might compare to the more like perspective of the scholar; on the contrary, it rejects the metahistorical deployment of ideal significations and indefinite teleology. It opposes itself to the search for origins' (Foucault 1977: 140). Following the preceding definition and explanation of the genealogical method, it will be instructive not to follow established metahistorical accounts but rather critically approach historical accounts of one or another place, event and birth of ideas. In this chapter I would like to go back to the beginnings or earlier practices of HIV disease and drug abuse.

To understand the dynamics of the evolution of the epidemic of HIV and drug abuse in Central Asia, it is useful to apply the genealogical method of Foucault to trace institutions, practices, culture, events, traditions, governance styles, control regimes, discursive formations, practices, textual and other linguistic events, verbal and non-verbal exchange, processes, historical developments, the background of the social, economic and political relations, and other important things related to the epidemic in question. The aforementioned method advanced by Foucault will enable me to look further into the Foucauldian biopolitics applied by national governments to address the epidemic in the country. Biopolitics is fundamental to national health policies in the region to which I will come back later.

M. Turaeva, *Drugs and Public Health in Post-Soviet Central Asia*,
SpringerBriefs in Public Health, https://doi.org/10.1007/978-3-031-09703-4_2

To make use of this approach to explaining drug abuse in the region, I conducted spatial, temporal and social spatial analyses of the evolution of drug abuse from pre-Soviet to Soviet to post-Soviet periods and went back and forth following social status systems and political engineering of the Soviets' contribution to the changing hermeneutics of the status of a drug user. Historical and political trajectories related to drug abuse and other health related problems are important and widely considered in the book. Following genealogical approach and ethnographic qualitative ethodology I traced drug abuse focusing on the relations between drug consumption and HIV as well as social embededness of behavioural patterns among drug users in the region.

2.1   History of Drug Consumption

Most Russian and Soviet authors speculate that the introduction of opium to Central Asia was initially made by Indian traders travelling across the Silk Road, which extended from south-west to north-east Uzbekistan connecting the historical cities of Khiva, Bukhara and Kokand. The time of extensive opium abuse ceased with Russian conquest in the second half of the eighteenth century, but local leaders remained in power until the October Revolution in 1917. As part of a colonial project, the region was widely explored by Russian scholars (Dobrosmuslov 1912; Semenov-Tyan-Shanskiy and Lamansky 1913). According to Antsiferov (1934), the centres of drug distribution in Central Asia were the Bukhara Emirate, the Kokand *khanate* and the Khiva *khanate*. Russian scholars (Tumanovich 1936; Ostroumov 1908; Shishov 1915) mentioned the consumption of *teryak* (opium) among the indigenous population of Central Asia as part of traditional food consumption and as part of healing practices which continue to the present day. According to Semenov-Tian'-Shanskiy and Lamansky (1913:4524), poppy was cultivated as an agricultural plant in Turkestan. From poppy seed people obtained oil and, moreover, extracted opium from poppy heads, and the rest was used for a narcotic beverage known as *kuknor*. The production of poppies increased in the region after the ban on opium production in China in 1729, and they were smuggled from India (Shishov 1915: 183) into Turkestan.[1] The smoking of opium was less prevalent in the region, but the main consumption method was to drink it after diluting the opium or parts of the opium plant (mainly capsules) in a watery solution. The smoking of hashish (hashish is a compressed resin gland collected from the unfertilized buds of the cannabis plant), drinking *kuknor,* especially in gambling houses or *Chayhona*[2] and

---

[1] The Turkestan region formerly included all Central Asian countries.

[2] *Chayhona* is a teahouse, where usually men gather to drink tea, play chess and cards, and eat the traditional Uzbek food *plov*. Chayhona still exists today. It is patronized mainly by men, who play games, watch TV, or simply eat *plov* and catch up on the recent local gossip in the neighbourhood.

other brothels, and entertainment with *bachas*[3] were mainly oriented towards male clients (Shishov 1915:454) in Turkestan.

According to Antsiferov (1929), a physician in a psychiatric clinic in Central Asia, in the pre-revolutionary Uzbekistan region, 4 out of 100 patients in psychiatric hospitals were dependent on cannabis (hashish). Antsiferov (1923) claimed that hashish and opium smoking was very widespread in Turkestan where hashish could be bought in teahouses. The well-known drawing *Opiumoedu* (The Opium Eaters) by Vasily Vereshchagin (1842–1904), a famous Russian battle painter who also accompanied Russian conquerors in Central Asia, shows the poor condition of people addicted to opium , for instance, their apathetic behavior.

2.2   Beginnings of the Punitive Methods to Address Drug Abuse

During Stalin's Great Terror, repressive measures were introduced to fight substance abuse with punitive methods, which drove drug consumption underground since drug users were treated as criminals (Latypov 2011b). In 1936, the Soviets claimed that 'social' illnesses such as drug dependence were supposedly eliminated from Soviet citizens' lives (Latypov 2012) due to the government's 'sanitary and enlightenment activities, conditions of the new *byt* [lifestyle] in kolkhozes, and *kul'turnost'* [cultured behaviour] of kolkhoz workers' (Fetisov 1937), which was politically prescribed. Publications of the time on drug abuse had an ideological character and was part of the aforementioned campaign against '*tuneyadzy*' (a type of societal parasites) also using these themes in accordance with the Cold War and the tendency to blame the West and capitalism for social ills (Latypov 2012; Gabiani 1990). Later Soviet medical literature on substance abuse mainly focused on alcoholism. Several decades of denying the presence of narcomania and toxicomania in Soviet Union led to a great dearth of knowledge and awareness about this problem. In 1974 in Soviet Uzbekistan, the sowing of opium poppies by the state for the production of raw materials in the pharmaceutical production of morphine, codeine and other opium alkaloids was prohibited (Kalachev, 1988). Some authors argued that the failed war waged by the Soviet Union (1979–1989) against Afghanistan resulted in a great influx of cheap drugs into the Soviet Union, smuggled through the porous Afghan borders. According to Kalachev (1989), Afghan War veterans (soldiers were recruited from all over the Soviet Union), who had seen their alcohol supply cut off,

---

[3] *Bacha* were young boys and adolescents who danced, sang in the company of men, and offered sexual services. *Bachchabozlik* (entertainment with young boys) was banned after 1922. According to Dobrosmuslov (1912:325), despite the female prostitutes (in Turkestan), there were also many *bachas* (male prostitutes), whereas all rich *sarts* (general term for all the settled natives of Turkestan used by Russians in nineteenth century) had their own *bachas* and those who could afford to keep a *bacha* paid a certain amount of money to his parents. Author (ibid) concluded by saying that one could find *bachas* in every teahouse.

switched to narcotics in Afghanistan. Some of them grew severely dependent when they returned home (Kalachev 1989, 1990).

In 1984 in the Soviet Union, operation '*cherny mak*' (black poppy) was launched, and opium cultivation and production were targeted for eradication. In 1986, there was less censorship and greater freedom of information under *perestroika* of Gorbachev in the Soviet Union. The topic of narcotics in the USSR and in Central Asia re-emerged in public discourse (in terms of recognition and removing the taboo on the subject), resulting in publications, newspaper articles, and so forth shedding some light on the situation of drug abuse. According to Ahmedov and Kadurov (1989:22–23), substance abuse spread because medical institutions, storehouses and chemistry-pharmaceutical enterprises were not provided with adequate security facilities. Thus, narcotics were easily stolen by workers or health professionals (see also Kilichev 1988:39), as were narcotic plants from kolkhoz fields which were used to satisfy demand for medical and scientific needs (Kalachev 1988). According to a retired man from Karakalpakstan (Kazakbedgoray, male, age 68, 2010) during the Soviet period, *kuknor*, a '*strong tea*', *was* basically consumed by old people who were over 70 years old in the region. *Kuknor* is a tincture or broth of opium poppy. The drink *kuknor*, which is basically tea made from plant opium poppy, is described to this day as a magic drink and is regarded as an ancient traditional remedy against all kinds of illnesses, such as headaches, rheumatism, back pain, and toothache, among many others. After drinking *kuknor* a person can easily work in the garden and doing household chores. *Kuknor* not only brings on a state of euphoria (*kayip*) but also restores a person's capacity to work. It was also stated in interviews that a small amount of opium was given to children suffering from diarrhoea, toothache and insomnia. The local habit of drinking *kuknor* was tolerated by the Soviet government because it was only done by retirees older than 70 years. A generational divide, which was a cultural phenomenon of local Uzbek communities, enabled the isolation of certain groups and their drug consumption practices. Drug consumption within a certain age group (elderly) was not seen as something negative within the community and attitudes towards it were relaxed, under the guise of 'letting them enjoy their old age'.[4] Many of my older informants confirmed this practice and also had similar views about drug consumption and age.

According to Kazakbay (Kazakbay, male, 74, 2010) *uchastkovy* (district) police knew about retirees who had cultivated opium poppy in their gardens. This was tolerated only for private consumption, not for selling. Others also established much bigger plantations to sell opium in Turkmenistan because opium use there was more common, so the market was also bigger. In Soviet times and after independence, there were no border controls between Uzbekistan and Turkmenistan up to 1994 (Zelichenko 2003). Taxi drivers usually delivered *teryak* (opium) to Turkmen consumers from the Karakalpakstan region in north-west Uzbekistan (Kazakbay, male, 74, 2010).

---

[4] Personal Communication, December 2010.

So far, I have tried to share some important and meaningful historical facts, discourses, and architectural and spatial denotations of some opioid plants, healing practices from very different times and diverse sources, such as literary sources, oral recollections, archival materials and historical media sources, among others, to give more space for diverse sources to avoid one-sided view of things. In what follows, I will continue to highlight some important recollections relevant to tracing the genealogy of epidemics of drug abuse in Central Asia, focusing on Uzbekistan.

2.3   From Bangi to Narkoman

Following the break-up of the Soviet Union in the early 1990s, there was a generational change in drug consumption patterns in Central Asia. By 1999, drug abuse had become a major problem due to drug abuse by young people, who enjoyed a wider availability of drugs at affordable prices (1 g of opium cost 40 sum, which was at that time cheaper than vodka, which cost 45 sum). According to Ahmedov and Kadurov (1989: 22), social conditions facilitated the epidemic of drug dependence in Central Asia. As a heritage of the past coupled with established traditional healing of many diseases using heavy drugs, the problem of mass drug abuse by youth also brought other social and public health issues (considering the large proportion of youth within the population). Edgor commented on and described this time as follows:

> Most of our generation without exception became dependent on drugs, everyone I knew became a drug addict, but at that time we didn't know much about it [drug abuse] and our grandfathers drank kuknor [his grandfather also consumed kuknor and planted opium poppies for himself], and there was nothing bad about it, and everybody respected them as *bangi* (Edgor, male, age 39, 2011).[5]

The social legitimacy of smoking opium (1980s to around 1995) due to the involvement of members of the upper class defined the status of *bangi*, which changed to *narkoman*, the term introduced by the state that carried a negative connotation, similar to criminal. Whereas the status of *bangi* was appreciated and valued, the transformation of the respectable name into that of a shameful category introduced by the Soviet state was inevitable. The transformation of the category of *bangi* to *narkoman* was a very slow process, and the two terms co-existed during the late Soviet times up to 1991, when the Soviet Union fell. The drastic change from *bangi* to *narkoman* happened when drug abuse by the younger generation became a mass phenomenon and a serious problem in the early 1990s to the early 2000s. After the break-up of the Soviet Union the borders became porous and not well guarded, drug routes were re-established, and economic migration started to gain momentum. The two developments which were relevant for the epidemiological condition of the region regarding drug abuse and increasing HIV infection were increased

---

[5] Interview October 2011.

migration (millions of migrant labourers and seasonal migrants between Central Asia and Russia) and the weakening of security along Afghan borders.

2.4   Genealogy of the Relationship Between HIV and STI

It is essential to look at the co-epidemiology of HIV and sexually transmitted infections (STIs) in the context of Uzbekistan, where there are alarmingly high rates of STIs among risky groups as well as the general population. Here it is important to go back to traditional healing practices which are locally more trusted because everyone's grandmother used them and lived to 80 years of age and older. Healing practices, religious healing and self-treatment with modern medicine are widely practiced. Self-treatment with modern medication is more recent than traditional healing practices, where religion and other beliefs play a role. Self-treatment became more and more popular with the introduction of the Soviet medical approach of injecting everything including vitamins. It is a common practice that medical doctors prescribe for minor health problems for both children and adults heavy medications and largely in form of injections. Otherwise doctors are also not taken seriously without such prescriptions which is locally known as *polnoe lechenie* ('full treatment' from Russian). The standard *polnoe lechenie* or a package of treatment would include 10 injections of antibiotics followed by 10 injections of vitamins (very bitter injections I must say as a child who grew up with vitamin injections). To be able to go for 20 injections to the polyclinic was not so easy, and each street or neighbourhood had a young woman or even a younger teenager (I myself was a self-made street nurse in my street in Urgench) who would perform all the injections on the residents in the same street or even neighbourhood in rural areas. Self-treatment was a result of these self-learned practices of injecting antibiotics and vitamins in local communities. Self-treatment for common illnesses was one thing; self-treatment for diseases which needed to be kept secret even from medical doctors was another. This was for instance true for STIs among women because the stigma related to STIs is usually gender biased and women with STIs are under much more pressure than men. Traditional restrictions on sex without marriage are another major issue which forces patients outside the state health care system to avoid stigma and grave social consequences, especially for women. CSWs and self-treatment are very popular, among PWIDs (male and female) and others. Information about self-treatment is shared among peers of the same group (CSWs, drug users). If no information is shared or available, the belief that taking any kind of antibiotic can help is widespread. Medical help is sought only in cases where self-treatment does not bring results.[6] A female drug user explained to me why one would not seek professional help when one has an STI:

> Have you yourself ever been to a dermovenereologic dispensary? Why go there? There is nothing there. What kind of treatment are you talking about, to go there only to figure out which antibiotic is needed and confirm you have syphilis? And then get registered (*na uchy-*

---

[6] Personal communication, AIDS clinic representative, December 2010.

ote)? ... No thanks ... I can figure that out even without going there (Rayhon, female, age 34, 2010).[7]

These and other factors make the prevalence of STIs a major problem which is also connected to the epidemic of HIV infection. Why is it important also to look at the presence of STIs while researchers investigate the main risky behavioural and injecting practices related to the transmission of HIV? The presence of STIs makes patients susceptible to contracting HIV compared to individuals without STIs. Some STIs can cause ulcers in vaginal mucosal tissue that can ease the transmission of virus to the bloodstream through the disrupted skin and mucous membrane barriers (USAID 2001). Many people who inject drugs (PWIDs) who engage in sex work are adolescents from Uzbekistan. Many sexually transmitted diseases are asymptomatic, and seeking treatment can be delayed, which means the virus can be transmitted to partners and clients without prior knowledge of the presence of infection. The system for monitoring STIs in Uzbekistan (I come back to the system of *uchyot* later in this book) is very poor and there are no available or reliable statistics on STI incidence, which makes it difficult to paint a true picture of the problem. This is also directly related to the general attitude towards STIs, which are viewed as something to be ashamed of, so people are reluctant to seek professional help. As for sex workers themselves, they are afraid of being locked in the clinics and finding themselves on the blacklists of *uchyot*. I will present the institution of *uchyot* later, in Chap. 3.

References

Ahmedov G, Kadurov M. Narkomaniya Prestupnost Otvetstvenost (Narcomania crime responsibility). Tashkent, Uzbekistan; 1989.

Antsiferov LV. Gashishizm v Turkestane i psikhozu v svyazi s num. Turkestankiyi meditsinskii zhurnal. 1923.

Antsiferov LV. Hashishism (anashism) in Turkestan. Proceedings of the First All-Union Congress of Neuropathologists and Psychiatrists. 1929. p. 40–41.

Antsiferov LV. Gashishizm v Sentralnoy Azii [Hashishism in Central Asia]. Tashkent; 1934. p. 45.

Dobrosmuslov AI. Tashkent v proshlom I nastoyashem [Tashkent in past and present]. Tashkent; 1912.

Fetisov GK. K Voprosu ob Anashakurenii (To issue about cannabis smoking). Za Sotsialisticheskoe Zdravookhranenie Uzbekistan. 1937;11(12):102–3.

Foucault M. Nietzsche, genealogy, history. In: Bouchard DF, editor. Language, counter-memory, practice. Selected essays and interviews, vol. 140. Itaca: Cornell University Press; 1977.

Gabiani AA. Na kraju propasti:narkomanija i narkomanu [At edge of precipice: narcomania and drug addict]. Moscow, Musl; 1990.

Kalachev BF. Drugs in Russia. Available in: http://narkotiki.ru/research_5283.html. 1988.

Kalachev BF. Narkotiki v armii [Drugs in army]. Sotsiologicheskie issledovaniya [Sociological research]. 1989;4:56–61.

Kalachev BF. Drug addicts in uniform. Sobyriya i Vremya. 1990;2:23–4.

---

[7] Interview, December 2010.

Kilichev F. Giehvandlik Jinoyatga boshlidi [Drug addiction lead to crime]. Tashkent, Mehnat [Labour]; 1988.

Latypov A. The administration of addiction: the politics of medicine and Opite use in Soviet Tajikistan, 1924–1958. PhD dissertation, University College London; 2011a.

Latypov A. The Soviet doctor and the treatment of drug addiction: "a difficult and most ungracious task". Harm Reduct J. 2011b;8:32.

Latypov A. On the road to "H": narcotic drugs in Soviet Central Asia. Central Asia Research Paper. 2012.

Ostroumov IP. Sartu. Etnograficheskiy materialu [Sarts. Ethnographical marerials]. Sredneasiatskay jizn. Tashkent; 1908.

Semenov-Tian'-Shanskiy P, Lamansky VI. Rossiya. Polnoe Geograficheskoe Opisanie nashego otechestva [Russia. The Complete Geographical Description of Our Fatherland]. Vol. 12. A.F. Devriena. Turkestanskiy kray. St. Peterburg; 1913.

Shishov A. Sartu. Ethnograficheskoe i antropologicheskoe issledovanie [Sarts. Enthnographic and anthropological research]. Tashkent; 1915.

Tumanovich O. Turkmenistan i Turkmenu [Turkmenistan and Turkmens]. Ashgabat: Turkmenskoe Gosudarstvennoe izdatelstvo; 1936.

USAID. Sexually transmitted infections, a strategic framework. United States Agency for International Development (USAID); 2001.

Zelichenko A. Istoriya afganskoy narkoekspansii 1990h [History of Afgan drug expansion in 1990th]. 2003. http://lib.ru/MEMUARY/AFGAN/afgan_drugs.txt_with-big-pictures.html. Accessed on 25 June 2013.

Chapter 3
Biopolitics of Foucault in Post-Soviet Central Asia

Health problems, such as drug dependence, tuberculosis, cancer, mental health, endocrine disruptors and occupational conditions classified as 'socially significant and hazardous', are being monitored closely by public health and security officials. In the context of post-Soviet states where Soviet-style governance remains in place and particularly when looking at health administration and management, it is striking that Foucault's theories of biopolitics and biopower, which go back to eighteenth-century Europe, can be easily applied to explain the health policies in the region. In the Soviet style of strict management of public health, punitive measures were very popular and constituted the foundation of the institutional basis of public health. This system consisted of healthcare units, security and forced labour units, which worked closely under the strict supervision of the Ministry of Internal Affairs. Forced labour was organized in the form of *lechebno-trudovaya profilaktika* (LTPs), which were labour correction camps for substance abusers. In a moment I will introduce these camps. Surveillance is ensured through the registration and blacklisting system of *uchyot*. To understand how health care is managed and regulated in Central Asia, it would be useful to draw on the framework of Foucault's biopolitics to analyse health management practices in the post-Soviet context. Biopolitics refers to the policing of bodies; thus, it is almost impossible in the context of an authoritarian regime to use the word 'care' at all. So instead of using health care, it would better to use health management or, even better, Foucault's term biopolitics. Biopower or biopolitics was explained by Foucault as 'a number of phenomena that seem to me to be quite significant, namely, the set of mechanisms through which the basic biological features of the species became the object of a political strategy, of a general strategy of power, or, in other words, how, starting from the eighteenth century, modern Western societies took on board the fundamental biological fact

Parts of the material in this chapter were previously published in Turaeva M, Turaeva R. Uchyot and Foucault: drug users and migration in Uzbekistan. Cent Asian Aff. 2021;8:83–98. https://doi.org/10.30965/22142290-bja10014.

that human beings are a species. This is roughly what I have called bio-power' (Foucault 1978: 1). Throughout his works on psychiatry, sexuality, punishment and discipline, Foucault reminds us about power over bodies and policing bodies. Foucault's interest in the architecture of the power of control and his famous panopticons is an impressive example showing how the field of architecture is integrated into these systems of power regimes. Authoritarian governments offer the best examples for applying Foucauldian concepts and theories.

Agamben (1998: 6) explained the 'intersection between the juridic-institutional and biopolitical models of power'. He (ibid.) argues that these two important aspects of power should not be separated and 'the inclusion of bare life in the political realm constitutes the original – if concealed – nucleus of sovereign power. It can even be said that the production of a biopolitical body is the original activity of sovereign power. In this sense, biopolitics is at least as old as the sovereign exception.' Explaining biopolitics and drawing largely on the works of Foucault, Agamben (1998: 6) states: 'Placing biological life at the centre of its calculations, the modern State therefore does nothing other than bring to light the secret tie uniting power and bare life, thereby reaffirming the bond (derived from tenacious correspondence between the modern and the archaic which one encounters in the most diverse spheres) between modern power and the most immemorial of the arcana empire.'

In what follows I will introduce an institutional setup of this system focusing on the institutions related to drug abuse and HIV/AIDS in Central Asia. In addressing public health problems, post-Soviet governments have applied Soviet tools to manage these problems. State and popular negative attitudes towards drug abuse, sex work, homosexuality, and HIV/AIDS and other contagious diseases stem from the Soviet ideology of creating a clean healthy Homo Sovieticus (Gogin 2012).

The aforementioned health problems and certain groups of people, like commercial sex workers (CSWs), have been put together in one pot to be cleaned, corrected, eradicated and punished. This kind of cleansing, correcting and punishing was done and is still done by means of strict control of the behaviour, forced medical treatment and registration system shared mutually within medical, security and other systems which are known as an institution of *uchyot*. This kind of strict punitive and forced approach, which is in use to the present day, I argue, does not contribute to the solution of the problems I address in this book. The main theoretical argument is that the institutional arrangement of the field of health management instead of health care implies the aim of the system is not to care for patients but to punish and control the unwanted parts of the population, such as drug users, sex workers, HIV-infected persons and other patients with infectious diseases.

The system of controlling unwanted behaviour, such as alcoholism and drug use, was strictly institutionalized. According to Babayan and Gonopolskiy (1990: 57), the social, medical and security fields closely cooperate to control unwanted behaviour. For instance, each enterprise has a drug control department which is linked to the Ministry of Internal Affairs.

In what follows, I will explain in detail how this system functions in order to control and punish bodies as opposed to delivering health care for citizens. Citizens are not seen as individuals with civil rights but rather bodies upon which biopolitics needs to be performed to keep the nation safe. A similar line of argumentation was developed by Agamben and his idea of Homo Sacer, where he explains that individuals first had their identity papers taken away so that their bodies, or 'bare life', could be acted upon where a human being without his official and civic papers is nothing more than flesh and soul. Agamben uses the example of Nazi concentration camps, where Jews and others were exploited and killed but after the victims had been deprived of their civil rights and were numbered instead. The system of public health control and control of risk groups includes clinics (both forced and voluntary), organizations both state and so-called non-state, which are in reality state organizations such as *mahalla*, which oversees all individuals belonging to a *mahalla*. The system also includes a registration system called *uchyot*, which is basically a blacklisting system shared within all state and non-state entities that have anything to do with patients or persons engaging in risky behaviours. Punishment and forced corrective labour are an important part of biopolitics. Punitive measures include but are not limited to imprisonment, constant police surveillance (raids) of those who are on the 'registered list' (*uchyot*, usually drug dependence is registered in medical institutions such as narcology centres, police stations, *mahalla*).

3.1   *Uchyot* – Main Tool of Biopolitics

There are special lists for people considered troublesome. These lists are maintained and shared by both medical staff and law enforcement and sit in one computer database. Before the advent of the computer the lists were shared in paper form. How is one entered in this system? Drug users can be entered into the system by being summoned to the police or by coming into contact with a narcological dispensary (*uchyotda*). People who inject drugs (PWIDs) who can afford treatment in private facilities are not registered, although one can never know. These lists are used for several purposes. According to a narcologist from Urgench, patients who are dependent on drugs or alcohol are usually registered (*uchyot*) in medical institutions for 3 years. As part of the system of *uchyot* narcology clinics where patients received treatment, doctors are obliged to continue visiting their former patients periodically to check on their patients after they return home. I was told that doctors, with their miserable salaries ($25 a month), cannot afford those visits but still are obliged to report that they perform those visits. *Mahalla* (neighbourhood) committees also have copies of this list, and their role within this system is to influence families and the target person to make sure that the targets behave well. Neighbourhood committees actively work in cooperation with both police and narcology clinics to help track those who are on the lists. There was one incident I came to know about in a particular neighbourhood during my fieldwork in 2011. One of the workers from the *mahalla* committee told his family he had a drug dependence, and he shared this with some neighbours, who then spread the news further. The drug user had just been released from a narcology clinic and was publicly declared to be someone who had gone to work in Russia. The case ended up with the drug user becoming violent towards members of the *mahalla* committee who spread the actual announcement around the neighbourhood.

To be removed from the list (after a minimum of 3 years), a registered patient following release from a narcology centre must prove steady remission. The proof will be presented by a formal procedure in which certificates are issued from the *mahalla* (neighbourhood) committee, *uchastkovy* (neighbourhood) police, and *uchastkovy* (neighbourhood) doctor; then the person can be removed from the blacklist of *uchyot*. Other ways or reasons for being deleted from the list are as follows:

- Change of residence to outside the territory served by the narcology institution
- Imprisonment for a term longer than 1 year
- Death
- Buying oneself off the list

Regarding the last item, it is more expensive to buy oneself off the *uchyot* than to pay a bribe not to register. Those PWIDs (who can afford to pay) who wish to avoid *uchyot* (registration) as a drug user in the database pay significantly higher fees at the few private clinics which provide private treatment (Wolfe et al. 2008). Therefore, often those who have the financial means pay bribes from the very beginning not to be entered into the system. The money received from patients is the main income of the working staff of the *uchyot* system, such as doctors of narcology centres and clinics, police and other places where the first contact took place. Everybody, including the family members of the victims, harbour great fears over being put on those lists since the price to get out is very high. Among the many consequences of being registered under those lists are losing one's driver's license, parental rights, the right to employment and admission to higher education, the right to marry and enforced 'collaboration' with law enforcement agencies. Drug dependents are not allowed to work in certain occupations. For instance, certificates stating that one is not listed in the *uchyot* system are part of the required list of documents to be submitted to register one's marriage. The list of documents also includes medical certificates indicating if one is healthy (no STIs) and HIV negative.

Soviet politicians designed the system of *uchyot* hoping to have a coordinated system of strict control over the risky behaviour of unwanted groups of citizens. In practice, the system serves to bring officials, doctors and others additional income from bribes paid by the families of victims and the victims themselves, in addition allowing them to exercise power and authority over others. The consequence of such a system is that people who need treatment are isolated and controlled. The system also pushes drug users and others who are potential victims of the system into practicing the unsafe use of drugs, unsafe sex and other health risks. Penitentiaries are prisons, psychiatric clinics (narcology departments within psychiatric clinics; the narcology departments were part of psychiatric clinics before 2003), and narcology centres which have the form of clinics (therefore I prefer using the word clinic to refer to narcology centres). According to my informants, these penitentiary institutions are the best places to get information about drugs, where to purchase drugs, what others do, how to inject and so forth. Mashrip (male, age 34, 2010)[1] told me that he was brought to a psychiatric clinic by his family members to get treatment for his drug dependence. He explained that before entering the psychiatric clinic he smoked heroin, and when he was released, he 'was on the needle', i.e. he had switched from smoking to injection. He stated that one of the PWIDs brought heroin, but there wasn't enough to go around for all the inmates to smoke it, so everyone agreed (who were heroin smokers) to inject it.

3.1.1   Soviet Narcology

The system of narcology clinics in the former Soviet Union is a Soviet legacy, i.e. the principles of fighting substance abuse are from the Soviet era. Narcology is seen as a discipline, a field, an institution, and a regime which is a Soviet creation. Within this authoritarian narcology system drug users and alcoholics are kept within the facilities of the narcology system, which resembles a prison. Narcology clinics carry out blood purification, aversion therapy and forced labour (Gilinsky and Zobnev 1998; Rouse and Unnithan 1993). Before narcology clinics were established, PWIDs were treated in psychiatric clinics in a separate special department. According to Babayan (1988), the Ministry of Health of the USSR issued a precept (No. 1180, 26 December 1975) to include the nomenclature of a new medical title – district doctor psychiatrist-narcologist (*uchastkovy vrach psikhiatr-narkolog*). Medical institutes re-established internships in psychoneurology and programmes of continuing education for doctors in narcology. The specialization *doctor-narcologist* was established. In 1976, narcology dispensaries were included in the nomenclature of healthcare agencies (order of the Ministry of Health No. 131, 5 February 1976) (ibid.: 54). Organization of narcology services consisted of health institutions (i.e. narcology, psychoneurology) and an institute of the Ministry of Internal Affairs of the USSSR (Babayan and Gonopolskiy 1990: 54).

In Soviet times, pharmaceutical narcotic drugs were issued by special prescriptions by doctors and only for medical purposes, and special prescription blanks had serial numbers and were subjected to special registration and control (Babayan and Gonopolskiy 1990: 47).

In 1987, the first HIV cases were detected in Uzbekistan, and when drug users were identified as the main drivers of the HIV epidemic in Uzbekistan, then only isolated, punitive methods were applied to block off the 'normal population' from the 'abnormal', which could be seen through the history of the management of PWIDs and the 'treatment' given to drug-dependent persons. The attitude that rose in the Soviet Union remains the same within the narcology system of fighting drug users and alcoholism. As one narcologist said:

---

[1] Interview, November 2010.

> If it was up to me, I would send them all to build pyramids, as was done previously. They must all be treated only with a whip … it doesn't work otherwise, i.e. they are just idlers and blissing out, they can only think of kefing (getting high) , they consciously did this, they live only at others' expense and one should not babysit them [*syusyukatsya*].

Patients at the narcology clinics have several options for dealing with withdrawal symptoms. A forced method was mentioned by IDUs themselves, which they called *v sukhuyu* (coming out of withdrawal symptoms with very limited or without medical assistance), voluntarily receiving detoxification medication and without this therapy (*v suhuyu*) as was mentioned by the patients of the clinics. The whole institutional structure, along with its discourses and practices of addressing such problems as substance abuse, was created by Soviet authorities to punish, control and correct unwanted behaviour to heal healthy bodies who would be able to work for Soviet industry. Ideas about what constitutes a healthy body resembled Nazi ideas of ideal bodies and ideas of unwanted bodies. In the current medical and biopolitical field of post-Soviet states, these approaches and attitudes have not really changed. Some policies and administrative structures were renamed to make them look more neutral, if not democratic, but in essence or content, the attitudes remained the same.

3.1.2 Present Narcology System in Uzbekistan

The system described in relation to the Soviet Union in the preceding section continues to exist in Uzbekistan. The system is fully financed by the state under the Soviet style of a centralized system of health care (Semashko). The present narcology centres and clinics in Uzbekistan are structured primarily to provide detoxification for opiate users and alcoholics, and no harm reduction interventions are offered to reduce HIV and hepatitis among drug users. There is one Republican Narcology Centre, 16 narcological dispensaries, 3 narcology inpatient clinics, and 11 narcology units within mental hospitals in Uzbekistan (National Centre on Drug Control under the Cabinet of Ministers of the Republic of Uzbekistan 2012). Additionally, attached to governmental narcological centres and clinics are 18 private clinics. All patients seek help at state institutions or are brought there by family members are automatically entered into the system of *uchyot*.

Governmental narcology dispensaries have about 1812 beds to provide treatment for substance abuse (National Centre on Drug Control under the Cabinet of Ministers of the Republic of Uzbekistan 2012), which mostly consists of detoxification with partial rehabilitation. The number of beds or places to treat drug users is 60 times lower compared to the number of estimated drug users needing treatment (Boltaev 2004).

3.1.3   Narcology Clinics: Case Study Narcology 1

This narcology centre is located in a small region in a village (the closest large town has a population of 1,200,000) of a distant district of Uzbekistan. It is located at the main highway connecting the towns. This is the only narcology centre in the *oblast* (a district). It was founded during the Soviet period in the early 1980s.

Regional narcology centres and clinics outside the capital city have not changed their Soviet style format of punitive methods, which make them more like prisons than clinics. Although narcology centres and clinics were established outside of psychiatric clinics, the narcological departments within psychiatric clinics continue to function in service of PWIDs and alcoholics who develop psychological problems and suffer epileptic shocks, who are referred from a narcology centre to a psychiatric unit. In both institutions the measures and negative attitudes towards inmates remained the same. In the Soviet Union, drug users and alcoholics were 'treated' in psychiatric clinics since narcology clinics did not exist. In the district where I conducted my field research, treatment for substance abuse and alcoholism was conducted in psychiatric clinics until 1981. A narcology centre opened in 1981 as a regional narcology centre – a separate institution dealing with *narcomania* (drug abuse) and alcoholism. The district narcology centre consists of three departments:

- *majburiy* (compulsory department)
- Voluntary department
- Rehabilitation department (which should encompass psychotherapeutic methods, which had not yet been established at the time of the research)

The *majburiy* department is a department (the worst of all departments) where patients are sent as a result of court decisions or brought by police. These departments are always locked with metal doors and secured with three policemen under 24 h guard. The internal perception of this department is very negative, too 'wild', not only by medical personnel but also by the PWIDs themselves. The whole security arrangement around this department contributes to this perception. *Majburiy* treatment in this department may be assigned by the court or by the family members of the 'troublemaking' drug users. The reasons given to me for why drug users end up in this department were as follows: the persons assigned to this department are those who are a problem: (1) not only to public peace [security] but also to their families; (2) these people pose a threat to other people, – in particular physical violence against family members or others, morality and health of the population.

Mashrip,[2] a male former inmate of this department, is 40 years old. He was transferred to the rehabilitation department from a *majburiy* department because of his health problems. He needed to be operated on (appendicitis) and in the recovery phase was placed in the rehabilitation department of the centre. He remembers his time in the *majburiy* department and complained that the rules and conditions there

---

[2] Interview, October 2010.

were similar to those in a prison. Usually, patients from voluntary departments could 'get out' for certain times, where 'out' means just remaining in front of voluntary departments in the garden or to smoke outside. His memories of the department were not fond ones. He also stated that the conditions were so bad that one becomes even more violent there, and there is no chance to recover from drug addiction; on the contrary, you learn even more about drugs from the inmates there. He said:

> In such a place [narcology centre] one would never quit drugs, look, but the opposite, one will learn more about drugs. (Mashrip, male, age 34, 2010)[3]

The voluntary department is for those drug users who come on a voluntarily basis to seek treatment without a court decision. A voluntary department also has 50 beds, and detoxification is the main treatment. Inmates complain that the 'free' food provided by the clinic is almost inedible, and those who can afford or have a supportive family have to buy their own food. The only difference I notice between *majburiy* and a voluntary department is that doors are not guarded by the police but just locked. Although the department is called voluntary, the inmates/patients are not allowed to leave the facility without official permission. Inmates also claim that they came voluntarily, but in reality they were all brought by family members or, in the best case, were contacted and asked to come voluntarily under threat of force. I have been told in a personal conversation with a narcologist[4] that people in voluntary and rehabilitation departments are admitted into the clinic on an anonymous basis, which is doubtful.

The first 3 days is a narcology detoxification period. There is no programme designed for patients and free time is spent watching TV or just lying in bed and talking. The rehabilitation department is the next destination after medical treatment ends. The department is supposed to offer rehabilitation measures. I had the impression that only privileged persons were accepted in this department because of the better conditions compared to the voluntary and *majburiy* (compulsory) departments (with 10 beds). Based on personal communication with a narcologist after 15–20, days of detoxification one can be transferred to the rehabilitation department.[5] The other narcologist commented (interview, 2010)[6] that they decided themselves whether or not PWIDs are eligible to be transferred to the rehabilitation department. All doors of all the departments were locked and keys were with medical personnel. There is a room for table tennis which is always empty; the only person who played was the 5-years-old daughter of one of the female drug users who was a patient there.

To my inquiries about the services to drug users and their families the director of narcology made the following statement:

---

[3] Interview, November 2010.

[4] Personal communication, October 2010.

[5] Personal communication, November 2010.

[6] Mavlon, 33, November 2010.

They [authorities above us] only know to demand from us, but the salary is small, of course we know that social workers should go to the families of PWIDs and the employment agency and ask what are the PWIDs' needs and help them, but all these activities need to be financed, but this is not done by the state; they only demand from us without any financial support, and we know ourselves what works and what should be done but there is always need of funding.

Food for the clinic was self-organized, meaning it was brought by patients' families and cooked privately, often by the cleaning workers. According to narcologists, most PWIDs come to the narcology centre just for 'washing out' (i.e., reducing an elevated dose of drugs in their system) or 'clean', 'blood purification' of their bodies from heroin, as they would say. Some PWIDs said, 'I came voluntarily to the centre in order not to ruin my body.' Some explained their stay at the narcology centre by claiming to follow the advice of family members (e.g. parents, wife) to quit drugs. Some patients had been there for a longer time, such as 6 months. 'I got in trouble with some crimes and had to disappear for a while to be forgotten,' said Umid.[7]

Another informant, Ikbol (female, age 34, 2011),[8] used to work as a trader. She sold goods in the bazaar and had worked for some time in Russia. She had two children, a son and a daughter. Her husband died from an overdose. She lives in her mother's house (her father had died) with her mother and children. In 2000 she was imprisoned for letting people smoke and inject drugs in her house. After being released from prison she started to sell drugs. To the question of why she started up with drugs again she replied:

I was released and came back and needed again to stand up on my own feet. Here we have no other possibilities, you know, if you want to start again with bazaar you need money for an initial investment.

The financial burden of feeding her children and financing her drugs caused her to fall back on selling drugs. She said that she came to the clinic to disappear from the drug market. Ikbol[9] said that in the time of her being in the clinic her mother took her place selling drugs. Working in the drug market at the lower ranks of sales and being a female is risky as the chances of becoming a patsy are high. Although the police have deals with various drug lords, there is always a need to catch someone to bolster crime statistics and so police officers can get promotions.

Other patients in the clinic were on drugs such as Kodatset® tablets in large doses (Turaeva & Engmann 2012). Kodatset patients needed to decrease their doses since it became unaffordable and physically unbearable to take high doses. A daily dose of Kodatset® cost the same as heroin per day. The patients stated that initially Kodatset was cheaper to inject than heroin. Over time, the Kodatset dosages grew, reaching such high levels that it became as expensive as heroin. Katya started with marijuana, switched to opium, later to heroin and finally ended with Kodatset. She

---

[7] Interviews, Uzbekistan, Male, 30, November 2010.

[8] Interview, October 2011.

[9] Interview, October 2011.

wanted to quit heroin but ended up becoming addicted to Kodatset®. Her last dosage before admission to the narcology clinic was 300 tablets of Kodatset® tablets per day. Katya argued that she thought that she could get the same high from Kodatset® as heroin but at a lower price.

Many PWIDs in their interviews said that the detoxification treatment given by clinic personnel had negative side effects, such as, for instance, dependency on psychotropic substances. Certain substances used to support drug users to withdraw from their drugs, depending on the prices of various painkillers:

> Here they go about getting you off drugs in the wrong way, giving us medicine, which also leads to dependency, it's just that you go from being dependent on one drug to another. This is not how it should be. They fill you up with cofilin and other psychotropic drugs, so you can't sleep normally and have to start taking sleeping pills, but then you get addicted to them too. Then depression sets in. So how do you treat that? And this continues until you just fall back on what you started with [heroin]. (Ruslan, male, 31 age, 2011)[10]

This perceived hopelessness leads to a loss of trust in medicine and spread within their communities, which has grave consequences for future trust in the medical profession, not to mention the constant surveillance they have to put up with. One size fits all was never helpful, whether for defining drug abuse, fighting drug abuse, defining drug users, judging drug abuse, or what have you.

3.1.4 Case Study Narcology 2 (Capital)

The Republican Narcology Centre was established in October 2003 in the suburbs of a big city. Many forms of therapy are provided to drug users, alcoholics and toxicomaniacs at this clinic. Services include both medical and medical-psychological-social models. Although some modernization of the methods of service provision and medical care have been introduced to the centre, which I described for the capital city where UNDP had contributed some co-funding for such services as art therapy in the capital city narcology centre, the narcology centres outside of the capital city are not the same. The first phase of care comprises clinical laboratory research, medical detoxification, and physiotherapy, for example. Among other therapies, the second phase of rehabilitation for PWIDs and alcoholics include, for example, milieu therapy, art therapy (funded by UNDP), medical and psychological investigations and individual consultation.

In Uzbekistan, rehabilitation services have been approved since 2006 in the field of narcology. In 2008, Republican Narcology Centre's focal point of therapy shifted from merely medical to medico-social rehabilitation. Officially, state facilities and centres are state funded and free of charge for patients. However, my informants stated that they had to pay for admission and other services within the clinic. This excludes those who cannot afford admission, and those who do not pay cannot

---

[10] Interview, January 2011.

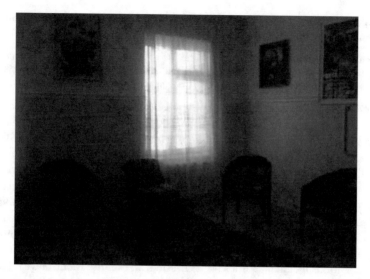

Fig. 3.1 Room for psychological therapy in rehabilitation departments

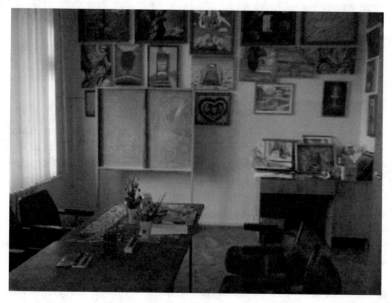

Fig. 3.2 Art therapy room. Drawings on the wall painted by patients. Art therapy is funded by UNDP

enjoy the services and medical help of the clinic. The chief of the rehabilitation department explained as follows:

> When a patient comes to the narcology centre, we offer him two options, firstly, a normal stay with daily [very basic] food, and the second option is better food, which the patient needs to pay extra for. This is in addition to the expenses from the government.[11]

Another representative of the narcology centre stated, 'The state does not have enough medication', which also should be paid for by the patients themselves.[12]

According to PWIDs, private narcology centres that perform only detoxification without psychological rehabilitation (Fig. 3.1) are very expensive. It should be noted that PWIDs who were in the rehabilitation department of Republican Narcology Centre were very satisfied with the services received and asserted that all services helped them recover from their drug dependency. Despite psychological training and art therapy (Fig. 3.2), patients have a very full daily schedule and are always busy with something (e.g. sports, therapy). Patients in the rehabilitation department are provided with better conditions in comparison to normal wards. These conditions include facilities for showering, an exercise room, and a recreation room with a TV; in addition, every room has its own toilets, among other amenities.

The narcology system of today in post-Soviet Central Asia is better than the past Soviet LTP system, although there are many similarities in approaches to dealing with drug abuse and attitudes of all involved, including personnel. Below I will outline the system of LTPs in order to shed light on the institutional setting of substance abuse in Central Asia.

3.2   LTP Camps Past and Present

Forced labour was designed to be part of corrective and punitive measures against unwanted parts of the population and risk groups. Corrective labour is also part of the prison system and was extremely harsh during Stalin's rule and his purges. The GULAG is an example of this system, where forced labour was extremely harshly imposed. The forced labour camps within prisons were called corrective colonies. Part of the corrective labour of a medical unit is organized in the form of LTP (*lechebno-trudovaya profilaktika*), literally translated as treatment-labour-prophylactic, meaning labour as both treatment and prophylactic. These camps used forced labour for all drug dependencies as a method to correct the risky behaviour of drug users during Soviet rule, and this could also be compared to corrective labour camps of post-socialist China for correcting Uyghurs' religion. In the latter it is ridiculous to define a religion as risky behaviour to be corrected. In the mid-1920s, many psychiatrists suggested treating drug-dependent persons and alcoholics with labour as an effective method. LTP colonies can be justifiably compared to

---

[11] Personal communication, October 2011.

[12] Interview, January 2010.

exploitation camps, where penal labour was applied. It has been argued that these types of institutions are not successful in their educational goals (Foucault 1995: 266).

The law On the Forced Treatment of Patients with Chronic Alcoholism, Addiction or Substance Abuse was adopted in 1992 under N 753-XII, and several amendments were made in 2000, with the most recent being in 2009. The law made changes in the terminology of the law on LTPs by changing the phrase 'medical institutions with special medical and labour regimes' to 'specialized treatment and prophylactic institutions of the system of the Ministry of Health of the Republic of Uzbekistan'.[13] Although the word labour has been deleted from the law, the LTP camps continue to function using old Soviet methods of corrective labour. In Turkmenistan laws on LTPs were not even changed and became even worse places according to one of today's LTP survivor stories I heard during my field visit in Turkmenistan in 2010. LTP camps function as colonies where chronic alcohol and drug abusers were usually forcibly admitted for 2 years without any prior commitment of crimes. The procedures of placement in these camps are regulated by the law on LTP camps. The procedures for placing drug users and other substance abusers are based on the recommendation of a narcologist and with a court decision. Complaints are often made by neighbours, colleagues, family members and others and the complaints are considered by local police. Narcological clinics can be a way to avoid LTP camps, but doctors can issue recommendations that a person be placed in an LTP camp. Initially, LTPs were created in the Soviet Union in the Kazak SSR in 1964. The first LTP camp in Uzbekistan was opened in 1987 in the Bukhara region. The LTP camp in the Khorezm region of Uzbekistan was established in 2003. LTP camps still function in most post-Soviet countries (Turkmenistan, Belarus and Prednistrovje) as well as post-Soviet Central Asia (only the names of the laws changed but the system remained the same).

The conditions under which drug users are 'treated' in the worst LTP camps are gruesome, such as those in Turkmenistan discussed in what follows. Farhod[14] (male, age 51, 2010) from Turkmenistan who was placed in an LTP camp four times. He explained that this place was worse than prison: 'people die there like flies', he said. Regular beatings (as part of treatment) and heavy work are the main methods of 'treating dependence'. Farhod's relatives didn't think he would survive his fourth 'treatment' visit in LTP. He explained that if he is sent again to LTP, he won't survive. In one of his dramatic stories from an LTP camp, a guard broke his leg hitting it with a metal shovel, and the wound opened and he received no medical help. Subsequently Farhod lay with his open wound for a month, only urinating on it in the hope that it would heal itself. He stated that drug users with no family support end up in LTP camps.

An Uzbek LTP camp opened in one of the Uzbek regions in 2003. Before this facility opened, drug users were sent to a neighbouring region. In each regional

---

[13] Available at: http://www.minzdrav.uz/documentation/detail.php?ID=1026.

[14] Interview in Turkmenistan, December 2010.

district, there is one district policeman who files complaints and brings drug users or alcoholics to the narcology centre for treatment. This is even more strictly practiced in Turkmenistan under very harsh conditions.[15] Representatives of the neighbourhood committees in Turkmenistan stated that there was a decrease in drug users since most of the drug users had been sent to LTP camps. The LTP colonies were financed from the profits of the labour of the inmates (drug users) working in the camp (Babayan and Gonopolskiy 1988: 69).[16]

What are other methods police use to catch drug users if there are no complaints or if complaints are made and the accused runs away? The police are very active in Uzbekistan, which is evident from their visibility in the streets, for example three to five policemen in each metro station and in the streets. Each *mahalla* (neighbourhood with two to three thousand flats) has a police department, and each district and regional unit has a larger police department. Drug users are very conscious of the intense police presence in their city and particularly in the capital city. Carrying syringes is also dangerous and can lead to arrest by police for drug abuse. Police conduct profiling not only in the metro and in the streets but also systematic home raids for illegal migrants, drug users and those involved in prostitution. Profiling of a drug user is easy and is based on a scrawny appearance and disheveled clothing. Drug users avoid public places, using metros and walking in the streets. All of the interviewees stated that they had been arrested at least once in their lives and been to prison.

3.3   New Methods with Old Rules: NEPs

The concept of 'harm reduction' was initially discussed in 1973, when the World Health Organization (WHO) Expert Committee on Drug Dependence acknowledged that traditional drug control measures did little to prevent drug use. The committee recommended additional measures to minimize 'the severity of problems associated with the non-medical use of dependence producing drugs' (WHO 1974).

Traditional harm reduction approaches include provision of sterile injecting equipment through needle exchange programmes (NEPs), community outreach to PWIDs and access to opioid substitution therapy. The governing principle of harm reduction is minimization of adverse consequences (in terms of health- HIV, HBV/HCV infections), social problems like joblessness and impoverishment from drug use. Stone and Shirley-Beavan (2018) reported that decreases in needle and syringe programme (NSP) site provisions have also been observed in Uzbekistan (last reported in 2016 from Global State of Harm Reduction), whereas in Kyrgyzstan, Tajikistan and Kazakhstan, provision of NSPs has remained stable. Turkmenistan does not have harm reduction programmes within the framework of any national

---

[15] An interview with a frequent patient of such a clinic in Turkmenistan, December 2010.

[16] More detailed information about LTP camps is given in a Human Rights Watch paper (1991: 55).

policies. Opiate substitution treatment (OST) is prohibited in Turkmenistan, Russia and Uzbekistan (Stone and Shirley-Beavan 2018). Methadone continues to be the most commonly prescribed substance where opioid agonist therapy (OAT) is available, followed by buprenorphine or buprenorphine naloxone (Harm Reduction International 2020).[17]

Evidence suggests that, to prevent the spread of HIV sustainably, NEPs need to reach more than 60% of drug users (Donoghoe et al. 2009). Some reports (Aceijas et al. 2007) indicated that less than 2% of PWIDs actually receive sterile injection equipment in Uzbekistan. The alarming incidence of HIV infection and drug abuse drew the attention of the international community, which resulted in funds being poured into 'harm reduction' programmes all over Central Asia. In Uzbekistan there was a network of 235 countrywide trust points (for needle exchange programmes) established to fight the HIV epidemic administered by an AIDS centre, at narcological dispensaries and polyclinics. Condom distribution for PWIDs and CSWs was also organized throughout the country. Huge amounts of funding for HIV programmes and other public health problems raised hope among funders and provided additional income for health managers but no hope for drug users themselves which can be heard from their comments on the new developments in the post-Soviet health system. PWIDs have limited or no access to prevention and health care services because of structural, legal and social barriers detailed in this book. Trust needs to be regained through health managers becoming health carers and security officers need to be taken out of the field of care before the target group can accept services. There are few harm reduction services provided for PWIDs with clean syringes and condoms outside the capital city. PWIDs mentioned that the number of clean needles was too small to 'waste one's time' going to the AIDS centre in a small town.[18] I will discuss here one of the NEPs in the form of an anonymous room but located in a polyclinic (a neighbourhood medical service unit for non-stationary treatment and diagnostics). The room was sponsored by international funding and coordinated with the AIDS centre. One of my informants (a drug user) commented on the new services as follows:

> Initially, when AIDS [SPID] came, nobody knew what it was, everywhere they started to distribute syringes, tea, condensed milk, *canned stewed meat*, and now there are so many cases of AIDS [in Uzbekistan]… they say 'Eegh, …here I recently wanted to obtain syringes but they [trust points] say they don't have any more … now they are used to AIDS cases and it's nothing new for them and it became normal for them because now there ae so many AIDS-infected people.' (Hakim, male, age 35, 2011)[19]

According to NEP workers, the location of NEP rooms in polyclinics successfully diminished the stigma of drug use and enabled PWIDs to enter and use the available services of NEP rooms without being identified as drug users. But after

---

[17] WHO has set NSP coverage target to 300 syringes per person who injects drugs per year to reach hepatitis elimination goals by 2030.

[18] Interview, October 2010.

[19] Interview, November 2010.

relocating this room from the first floor, where it was initially located, to the third floor, the number of PWIDs using services decreased. They believe that the reason for relocating the room from the first floor to the third floor was jealousy of the administration who could not stand the fact that the room for drug users was well equipped with such items as an air-conditioner and underwent renovation sponsored by the project, whereas other rooms and facilities for sick people and children of the neighbourhood were in a poor state. Another NEP room was located next to a local AIDS clinic. Not every PWID *dares* to enter the AIDS centre in order to obtain clean syringes. It is not acceptable if one is seen to be entering the territory of the AIDS centre since the stigma of being HIV infected has grave consequences; for example, it is worse to have AIDS than to be a drug user. Male drug users might still have hope that they can change their behaviour, whereas being infected with HIV leaves one entirely bereft of hope and in danger. Another informant commented on NEP rooms as follows:

> Whoever goes to these places [NEPs] for syringes would be *registered* [entered into the *uchyot* lists]. But who wants to *reveal oneself* as a *narkoman* [drug user]? If one lives, for example, in Sputnik [one of the neighbourhoods] and spends 500 sums for local transport to reach this room? For those 500 sum he could buy 10 syringes [a single syringe costs 50 sum in a drugstore], and even if he goes there when he somehow ends up downtown, he'll only get a few syringes and lots of *annoyed* looks. (Shurik, male, age 35, 2011)[20]

To the question 'do you have PWID clients regularly?', one NEP worker proudly showed me a registration book where all 'client' details were written accurately. I wondered about the anonymity principle of these new projects and service points. Another PWID stated:

> A drug dependent is a person who only thinks about money … in these new places [NEPs] they used to distribute 10 syringes and 10 condoms, and also before they used to distribute *canned stewed meat*, tea to each narcomaniac, and then what will such a narcomaniac do? He will go around in all these rooms and collect syringes from all possible places and gather them in one box – in a drugstore one syringe costs 100 sum – and he sells one for 50 sum to drug stores and makes money for heroin and also tea and other stuff he also sells in the bazaar. (Hakim, male, age 35, 2011)[21]

The main reason why most PWIDs prefer not to use NEP services is out of fear of being registered and being caught by police and the shame of entering such a place, which in their eyes is not worth the syringes. According to a national study under the auspices of the Ministry of Health of Uzbekistan with the support of UNODC (2006), PWIDs do not use the services of trust points because they are afraid of being caught by police and being registered (*uchyot*) or being seen by someone who knows them and might identify them as drug users. It is safe to say that the situation with general mistrust in any services offered by the state or non-state organizations remains the same, which was statistically proven in the afore-mentioned 2006 UNODC study. Current surveys are being conducted and hopefully

---

[20] Interview, October 2011.

[21] Interview, January 2011.

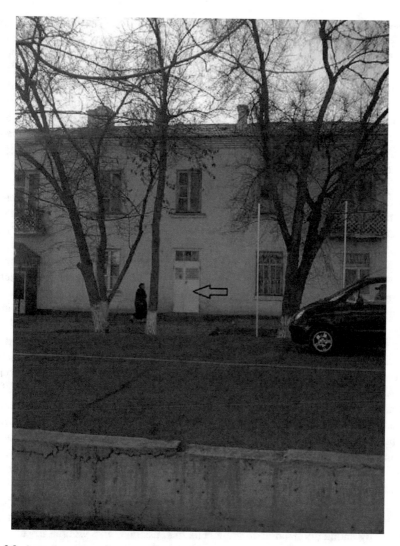

Fig. 3.3 Anonymous room in a town of an Uzbek district

new results on this important issue will be published soon. My most recent exchanges by mobile app with contacts from my field research also sounded as if things had not changed for the better at either location where I had conducted my fieldwork. The trust of the vulnerable populations discussed in this book needs to be earned considering local traditional cultural institutional settings, which are diverse not only within Central Asia but also within individual countries.

Another '*anonimnaya komnata*' (anonymous room) was located within a private flat of a family (Fig. 3.3). The room was supposed to provide information on HIV/ AIDS, STIs and reproductive health. Most times I tried to access the room it was closed, and once I was fortunate to find the room open. To my surprise I met a small boy playing computer games in the room and I had a short conversation with him to find out what the room was about and what he was doing there. The boy happened to be in his own home and the room was supposed to be a room for drug users to obtain information anonymously. The boy indicated that he was told to be there and was the person in charge of the room, according to the instructions of his mother, who was sleeping. The boy was also surprised that somebody had entered the room. The room was declared to be a non-governmental organization (NGO) involved in collaborative preventive projects to eliminate HIV/AIDS, STIs and drug dependence and provide information. Funding for the 'room' was received from the Ministry of Health, which I found out from the woman who was supposed to run the 'room'. 'Health' projects, and other health-related works, such as security, control and medical services, are housed under the Ministry of Health. Although the aforementioned NGO above was supposed to be non-governmental, funding came from the ministry.

In what follows, I will detail another encounter with the new methods put in place with the financial support of international donors. One of the directors (Reimbergan) of the narcology centre where I spent most of my time asked me to attend one of the meetings he did not want to attend, which was obviously obligatory. The meeting was organized by an NGO, which received a small grant (2 million som, around USD 800) to work with drug users. The NGO organized the meeting with members of the *Mahalla*[22] committee (neighbourhood committee), medical university, other NGOs, Kamolot (state youth organization and fund) and the AIDS centre. I was introduced as someone representing a narcology centre since I was accepted as an intern in the clinics where I spent most of my time. The director asked me to represent his narcology centre there and register the name of the centre in the participant list so that the centre was recognized as a participant. Obviously, having a presence at state-organized events for the relevant stakeholders is part of their work obligations, which are overseen by relevant institutions. Reimbergan explained to me that the grant was used for preventive and educational programmes to fight drug abuse and HIV/AIDS. The event took place in a very small café. During the event I came into contact with a man from a medical university which was funded by another collaborative grant. The man assigned me, without my consent, the task of presenting his slides on drug users for him. I refused his request, saying that I was unfamiliar with his topic well and that, furthermore, I was not in a position to present someone else's ideas. He became very angry with me and showed his disgust over the fact that a young girl like me had dared to refuse his order. Later I found out that this man was a high-ranking official from a medical university. There was no audience, but photos were taken, as if presentations had been made to an imaginary audience and laptops which did not function were displayed for service

[22] *Mahalla* – is a traditional social institution which is responsible for observing everyday people's lives and registering all members of a community in all matters regarding who had migrated where, what illness (alcoholics, drug users, mentally ill) they brought with them, and, in prison, who came from abroad, who is abroad, which families need social support, and so forth.

the object of the photo shooting session. The whole event seemed to be happening solely for the sake of holding the event because of grant reporting. Coffee, sweets and food were an attraction rather than the content of the event. No discussions were held, and no questions were asked in order to enable earlier end of the same event. I reported the event to the director of the centre who had sent me there, and he did not seem surprised based on past events he himself had attended. His comment was as follows:

> It is all *boltavnya* (twaddle) and all are keen on the pens which are distributed. […] Yes, people go to these events in order to get their free pens. The invitation to this event was made up nicely, and the aim of the seminar was said to be the 'Promotion of healthy lifestyles among the youth, prevention of drug abuse and HIV infections and AIDS and measures to fight these problems.'[23]

Novel approaches to address drug abuse largely introduced by international organisations have not always been accepted due to their failure to consider local mindset and other traditions. One of the most successful attempts at intervening with maximum consideration of the local context and the Soviet past was the Central Asia Drug Action Programme (CADAP), the results of which still need to be seen after systematic qualitative studies of the same problems I am considering in this book.

3.3.1 Project OST: Failed Efforts of Methadone Introduction

Opioid substitution therapy (OST) was established as a pilot project in the capital city in 2006, where buprenorphine and later methadone were given to HIV-positive drug users only. It was sponsored by the Global Fund and implemented in the Tashkent Narcology Dispensary wherein 271 patients were included (Kargin 2007). In 2006 Uzbekistan was the first country of the former Soviet republics to establish buprenorphine and methadone programmes, but only for HIV-positive patients, though later HIV-negative dependent patients were allowed as well. By November 2007, 90 patients were receiving buprenorphine and 37 methadone in Uzbekistan (IHRD 2008). However, Godinho et al. (2005) estimated that approximately 5% of PWIDs in Central Asia were covered by harm reduction programmes. In 2009, a pilot OST programme was shut down, and the Uzbek government refused to restart the programme, referring to its ineffectiveness despite WHO evaluation of the pilot project, which demonstrated positive trends for patients after the start of treatment, such as a decreased use of illegal drugs, improvements in general health and decrease in criminal activity (Michels et al. 2017).

Hakim (male, age 35, 2011),[24] who is HIV-positive and was treated in the narcology centre during my visit, explained to me his vision of the OST programme from

---

[23] Personal communication, October 2010.

[24] Interview, January 2011.

a drug user's perspective. He stated that many PWIDs had been exposed to methadone, which was 'brought out of the clinic'. Either they sell it or inject it themselves intravenously. Another informant who was in the OST project explained why pilot methadone therapy was unsuccessful in Tashkent:

> When you are on methadone you don't feel kef of heroin anymore, so it is a waste of heroin if you inject it after methadone, which is why many PWIDs somehow bring methadone out [of the dispensary] and sell it to buy heroin, and others buy methadone and dissolve it with Dimedrol® and inject the mixture to get kef. (Hakim, male, age 35, 2011)[25]

Hakim said that no one of those who were on heroin really wanted to quit drugs. Thus, being in a methadone programme represent another means of obtaining a drug in order to resell it and ultimately score some heroin. To the question of how one could bring methadone out of the dispensary, he replied:

> A drug dependent is a person who finds all kind of ways to get money … what I did is I stuck chewing gum on my upper jaw. When the doctor gives you tablets, you close your mouth and pretend to swallow but in fact you stick the tablet in the gum. Or when a doctor gives tablets to others (PWIDs), you distract her/his attention, and that is how methadone leaves the dispensary unnoticed. (Hakim, male, age 35, 2011)[26]

Many PWIDs heard about the methadone pilot project and the possibility of buying methadone tablets from unreliable patients. Denis (male, age 25, 2011), in response to a question regarding OST, expressed a negative attitude: 'This methadone they provide ruins all your teeth, just look at all narcomaniacs who were on this treatment, they all lost their teeth.'

The results of attempts by the OST pilot project to eliminate drugs from the clinic/centre were not exclusively negative; there was also positive feedback (e.g. Kargin 2007). The positive results of the OST pilot project were services, such as by psychologists, social support and access to friendly private rooms. Kargin (ibid.) showed improvements in physical conditions, finding jobs and re-establishing a family. Despite OST's clinical effectiveness and cost-effective drug treatment strategy, and despite the fact that it has been shown to substantially reduce drug-related crime and infectious diseases (HIV, Hep C) and support the effective treatment of other health problems and dependencies (Stoever et al. 2020; Sorensen and Copeland 2000; Gowing et al. 2004), OST is prohibited in Turkmenistan, Russia and Uzbekistan (Stone and Shirley-Beavan 2018).

3.3.2 Incarceration and Cleaning

The reason for not carrying syringes on one's person is the possibility of being arrested by the police on a random check. In Uzbekistan, as well as generally in Central Asia, one encounters police everywhere, not to mention the metro in the

---

[25] Interview, January 2011.

[26] Interview, January 2011.

capital city Tashkent, where four to six policemen guard each metro station. Police do maximal and continuous profiling in the hope of detaining the highest number of victims who will be willing to pay for their freedom. Profiling of drug users is very easy since drug users have notable physical features. Drug users must think twice about going to centres for new syringes or needles, so appearing in public spaces poses an additional risk to drug users, who try to avoid going to the centres at all costs. All of the interviewees stated that they had been arrested at least once in their lives and done prison time. Many of the interviewed PWIDs stated that had learned about drugs, e.g. what other drugs can be injected, what drugs to mix to get a stronger kef, criminal activities of other inmates, and how and where to make money in prisons. Many PWIDs mentioned that drugs were also available in prison, which is clearly not possible without the collaboration of prison authorities and other state actors as well. One of my informants made the following statement:

> In prison it [heroin] is openly sold. If you give the police money, they will bring it to you … so let's say, for example, 5 people pool their money for heroin and have only one syringe. All five will inject heroin with the one syringe. (Hakim, male, age 35, 2011)[27]

Obviously, some PWIDs who had no money were forced into involuntary abstinence. Overdose often occurred after long imprisonment when the drug user took heroin at the old dosage because the body's tolerance of the drug had already diminished. Knowledge about overdosing and why and how it happens is widespread nowadays among drug users based on their own experience and through interactions with their peers.

References

Aceijas C, Hickman M, Donoghoe MC, Burrows D, Stuikyte R. Access and coverage of needle and syringe programs (NSP) in Central and Eastern Europe and Central Asia. Addiction. 2007;102:1244–50.

Agamben G. Homo Sacer: sovereign power and bare life. Stanford: Stanford University Press; 1998.

Babayan EA. Narkomanii i toksamanii [Narcomania and Toksamania]. In: Morozova GV, editor. Guidelines on psychiatry. Moscow: Meditsina [Medicine]; 1988. p. 169–218.

Babayan EA, Gonopolskiy MH. Uchebnoe posobii po narkologii [Tutorial on narcology]. Tashkent Meditsina UzSSR; 1988.

Babayan EA, Gonopolskiy MH. Narkologiya [Narcology]. Moscow: Meditsina; 1990.

Boltaev A. Needs assessment on HIV and drug policy in central Asian countries, access to primary health care for drug users. Open Society Institute; 2004

Donoghoe M, Verster AD, Mathers B. WHO, UNODC, UNAIDS technical guide for countries to set targets for universal access to HIV prevention, treatment and care for injecting drug users. Geneva: WHO/UNODC/UNAIDS; 2009.

Foucault M. Security, territory, population: lectures at the College de France 1977–78. New York: Picador; 1978.

Foucault M. Discipline and punish. The birth of the prison. Vintage; 1995.

---

[27] Interview, January 2011.

Gilinsky Y, Zobnev V. The drug treatment system in Russia: past and present, problems and prospects. In: Klingemann H, Hunt G, editors. Drug treatment systems in an international perspective: drugs, demons, and delinquents. Thousand Oaks: Sage Publications; 1998. p. 117–23.

Godinho J, Renton A, Vinogradov V, Novotny T, Rivers MJ, Gotsadze G, Bravo M. Reversing the Tide: Priorities for HIV/AIDS Prevention in Central Asia. World Bank Working Paper No. 54. Washington, DC: World Bank. © World Bank. 2005. https://openknowledge.worldbank.org/handle/10986/7354 License: CC BY 3.0 IGO UNODC.

Gogin S. Homo Sovieticus: 20 years after the end of the Soviet Union. Russian Analytical Digest; 2012.

Gowing L, Farrell M, Bornemann R, Ali R. Substitution treatment of injecting opioid users for preventing transmission of HIV infection (Cochrane review protocol) Cochrane Library, Issue 3. Chichester: John Wiley and Sons Ltd; 2004.

Harm Reduction Developments 2008. New York: International Harm Reduction Development Program of the Open Society Institute.

Human Rights Watch (1991). Prison conditions in the Soviet Union. Human Rights Watch, New York. The Global State Of Harm Reduction 2020 7th Edition. Harm Reduction International. 2020. Available at: https://www.hri.global/files/2021/03/04/Global_State_HRI_2020_BOOK_FA_Web.pdf.

Kargin S. Substitution therapy pilot project: The first set of result. Power point presentation. 2007. http://www.powershow.com/view/12351b-OWYyM/Program_Scaling_up_the_Response_to_HIVAIDS_in_Uzbekistan_a_Focus_on_Vulnerable_Populations_under_th_flash_ppt_presentation. Accessed in 29 Feb 2012.

Michels II, Keizer B, Trautmann F, Stoever H, Robelló E. Improvement of Treatment of Drug use Disorders in Central Asia the contribution of the EU Central Asia Drug Action Programme (CADAP). J Addict Med Ther. 2017, 5(1): 1025.

Rouse TP, Unnithan NP. Comparative ideologies and alcoholism: the protestant and proletarian ethics. Soc Probl. 1993;40:213–27.

Sorensen JL, Copeland AL. Drug abuse treatment as an HIV prevention strategy: a review. Drug Alcohol Depend. 2000;59(1):17–31.

Stone K, Shirley-Beavan S. Global State of Harm Reduction 2018. Harm Reduction International: London.2018.

Stoever H, Michels II, Aizberg O, Boltaev A. Opioid Agonist Treatment for Opioid Use Disorder patients in Central Asia. Heroin Addiction and Related Clinical Problems. 2020.

Turaeva M, Engmann B. A new pattern of drug abuse among injecting drug users in Tashkent city. Journal of substance abuse.2012.

Wolfe D, Elovich R, Boltaev A, Pulatov D. HIV in Central Asia: Tajikistan, Uzbekistan and Kyrgyzstan. In: Celantano DD, Beyrer C, editors. Public health aspects of HIV/AIDS in low- and middle-income countries: epidemiology, prevention and care. Springer: New York; 2008. p. 557–81.

World Health Organization. WHO Expert Committee on Drug Dependence: Twentieth Report. World Health Organization; Geneva: 1974.

Chapter 4
Individual Concerns of Drug Users and Drug Consumption Patterns Among the Research Participants

4.1 Socio-Demographic Information

Although this study counts 50 official drug users, there were also others who were in friend circles, consuming or not consuming drugs, who I only met once. Therefore, only those who I followed systematically and interviewed appear in the analysis presented in this chapter. The following descriptive statistics will help to visualize the group to be able to show the situation in numbers. The total number of drug users interviewed was $n = 50$ (100%). Out of 50 drug users, 41 were male (82%) and 9 were female (18%). At the time of the interviews, the mean age was 35 years, the median age was 34.5 years, the youngest case was 20, the oldest 60 years old. Most of the informants were of Uzbek ethnicity (68%), followed by Russian (18%). The age of onset was mean age 17.5 years, median age 16, whereas the earliest initiation of drug abuse was at 14 years old and the latest at age 25 years. Officially employment prevailed among male drug users (22%) versus women (11.1%). Both male and female drug users dominated in the category 'other' when answering the question of employment. Most of the participants who answered the question about employment as 'other' are unemployed but nevertheless pursue some kind of economic activity locally referred to as '*biznes*', which means basically anything that brings some kind of income such as small-scale trade (mainly unofficial and illegal) or doing some cash-based labour in markets such as carrying bags. Most of my informants are discarded from society to survive shadow living. It is noteworthy that none of the drug users lived on the street or were homeless. Men more often lived in the household of their parents (65.9%) than women (33.3%). The data confirm the findings of a larger study where similar results were obtained for an earlier period with a sample size of $N = 1000$ drug users from Uzbekistan from 2006 in comparison with my own data from 2010.

Fifty percent of people who inject drugs (PWIDs) were married. Most of the male PWIDs were married (56.1%) and their wives had to bear a double financial and moral burden. The willingness of women to live with active PWIDs can be well explained by the high social pressure, wherein women who return to their parents' home (usually after domestic violence) are automatically be labelled prostitutes. The social and economic pressure on women who are reluctant to divorce, even if their husbands are active PWIDs, is the norm and additionally garners a kind of prestige for the women, who are respected for this tolerance. One ex-drug user's wife stated:

> … whatever husband it is I have to bear that, while leaving him and returning to the parents' house it won't be better, everyone will blame me and on top of that they will call me a prostitute, so I don't care, let him die soon, at least I will remain with shelter; otherwise I will have to return to my parents house and live on their expenses. Let's say I live with my parents one or two years; then I'll also be a parasite with my children.

4.2   Changing Patterns of Drug Consumption

Drug users from the capital city of Uzbekistan preferred cannabis (*anasha*). In the south-western part of Uzbekistan, a distant and smaller district, *kora dori* (opium) use prevailed. In the district of the capital city there is only one drug user who preferred *kora dori* (opium) as a gateway drug. There are differences between the north-east and south-west in terms of gateway drugs. In the north-eastern part, cannabis was the favoured gateway drug. In the south-western part (distant district), opium dominated. Possible causes of this might be the fact that opium was very widespread, available and cultivated in the district (south-western region). The data also show that there is a new trend towards cannabis narcomania in Uzbekistan among young people, which was also confirmed by medical personnel at narcological centres.

There are three categories of drug users, high-class (no local name, only description), middle-class (*bangi*) and low-class drug users (*shiroviye* or *konechenniye/* those who could not afford real drugs anymore). This categorization is emic. The high-class drug users differentiate themselves from all the other drug users as 'the cleverest' ones with good educations. What I call middle-class drug users, or *bangi* in the local term, are considered those drug users who can still afford to smoke heroin, in particular using a waterpipe constructed from plastic bottles (*bulbuly-ator*). I will detail all the methods and combinations shortly. What is referred as the lowest type of drug users or low-class users (*shiroviye* or *koncehniye*) are those who stopped injecting heroin and switched to cheaper versions of drugs such as, for example, injecting Kodatset. It is also known that those well-off drug users sell the rest of their 'smoked water' to the '*shirovy*' for a little money or give it away for free in return for some other favours, for example, manual labour in their homes or other services. The rest of the 'smoked water' is then evaporated (0.5 L is evaporated into one doses of injection amounting to 5 mL) by low-class drug users for injection, which can also be combined with Dimedrol (sleeping medication or anti-allergen).

Other methods of drug consumption are also associated with low-class drug users, such as using dirty, not boiled, water for injections, for example, using water from canals. This happens because there are no hidden spaces where they might have access to clean running water and electricity. Most drug users hide their drug consumption from their families and so must take drugs in secret. In contrast, more well-off drug users have more possibilities when it comes to space available for taking drugs, such as at home or even in separate flats where they can consume drugs freely without family members noticing it.

4.3   *Beshabashnoe* (Chaotic/Anarchic) Times

The early independence period was characterized by economic crisis coupled with the epidemic of drug abuse, resulting in a skyrocketing crime rate (Nazpary 2002). This period even saw the re-emergence of bazaars (*koyna bazaar*) where stolen items were bought and sold, with mainly PWIDs selling whatever they stole from their own families or other places in order to be able to buy drugs. Drug lords also introduced barter exchanges for drugs with any items brought by their clients in order to keep them as potential clients.

In 1989, in some Central Asian republics, a reported 70–80% of crimes were committed to obtain money for drugs (Davis 1994). The emergence of gang-like organizations, so-called drug mafias, was observed and drug cultivation became popular throughout Central Asian republics (Kuleshov 1990). The time was also perceived as one of new opportunities by informants who spoke about easy money, such as small-scale trade and easy robberies which went unpunished and a proliferation of scams (one PWID said he had developed a network of shell game (*'obman glaz'*)[1] conjurers at a bazaar. The proliferation of secret medical services privately 'treating' drug users also brought high profits to medical professionals.

4.4   Post-Soviet Patterns of Drug Abuse

The transition in drug consumption methods changed from smoking to risky injection methods due to the shortage of opium and heroin on the drug market. A drug shortage was caused by several factors, such as drug cultivation reduction in Afghanistan in 2000, tight regulation of drug sources and tighter border control (after independence of Uzbekistan). My own findings and those of others (Harris

---

[1] *Obman glaz* (optical illusion) games are similar to the shell game. Players have to guess which box a die is under. Three boxes are moved around very quickly, and every so often the conjurer quickly lifts up a box to reveal the location of the die and quickly pufs the box back down over the die, doing this several times so the spectator loses track of the die. Finally, the spectator has to guess which box the die is under. But it's always a trick.

et al. 2015) highlight the fact that there is a need for enhanced service provision during periods of drug shortages. Most of the transitions to harder drugs – such as from cannabis smoking to opium eating and drinking then smoking, from anasha (cannabis) to hashish, from opium injection to heroin injection, from heroin smoking to heroin injection, from heroin injection to heroin in combination with other substances, from heroin injection to other medicine (Kodatset) – in most cases occurred due to an increase in the cost of drugs, the impoverishment of drug users, an interest in trying something stronger, or forcible injection of drugs.

According to Oybek, the transition from sniffing heroin to injecting happened because friends who had always sniffed started to inject, so one was sniffing, the other injecting, and that lasted for a while (where those who started to inject kept saying it was better kef and cheaper) and at the end everybody would follow the 'innovator' (Oybek, male, age 38, 2010). Narcologists stated that with worsening economic conditions and the closing of borders they observed a shift from drug abuse to heavy alcohol abuse. Particularly economically impoverished PWIDs switched to alcohol and previous patients of drug abuse were becoming patients of alcohol abuse. Drug users saw alcohol abuse as much more visible than drug abuse. The argument against alcohol consumption was that drug consumption could be more easily hidden than alcohol. Social stigma and social pressure play a major role in the decision-making of PWIDs and their behaviour. Some PWIDs who switched to binge drinking combined it with smoking of cannabis as well. According to them, one matchbox of cannabis costs in Urgench 5000 sum (~2.5 euros) which is enough for one person to smoke for a week. Uzbekistan's capital Tashkent consists of 11 regions, and the price of drugs drops off substantially as one moves from the city into its outer regions. According to interviewed PWIDs, the price for heroin in Tashkent is in the range of 25,000–30,000 sum (~10 euros is one *chek*). But PWIDs also explained, 'If for example one even goes to the Kuyluk district of Tashkent, which is the last district of the city, and then drives 2 km further, the price drops to 15,000 sum (~5 euros); drive a bit more and the price becomes 10,000 sum (~3 euros)'. Accordingly, many PWIDs travel outside of Tashkent to get heroin. In other cities, the prices are lower than in the capital. In Khorezm one *chek* costs 20,000 sum (~6 euros), and 1 g is 80,000 sum (~26 euros).[2] Hakim (male, age 35, 2011)[3] explained that because the price differs so much, one might drive 50 km or even 100 km from Tashkent to buy heroin. Yangiyul, a small city 20 km from Tashkent with a population of 60,000, is considered one of the nodes of infection since 2000. As Tashkent residents explained, in early 2000 it became the main drug selling location. Drug users went to buy heroin and injected immediately with any available syringe at the point of purchase. They might pick one up from the street, borrow from an injecting partner, or even use a stranger's. Respondents explained that every household in one street at that time was selling drugs. One could find in each corner of a house a mountain of syringes left by PWIDs.

---

[2] Personal communication, Tashkent, January 2011.

[3] Interview, January 2011.

Before heroin was introduced to the region, the most common drugs in Uzbekistan had been marijuana and raw opium, which could be transformed by simple methods into a ready-for-use drug called *khanka*[4] (in the Khorezm region, it is called *teryak* or *kora dori*). Khanka still accounts for 79% of the drugs used in Uzbekistan, 75% in Almaty and 97% in Bishkek (Kyrgyzstan) and 90% in Tajikistan (Renton et al. 2006). Smoking marijuana continues to be fashionable among young people in Uzbekistan, but the mid-1990s marked a shift from smoking opium to the injection of homemade preparations of *khanka*.

4.4.1   Opium: Injection of Kora Dori (Opium)

The present methods of preparing opium for injection vary. During the Soviet period people used to inject opium in combination with acetic anhydride, which was widely available and purchased from creamery (personal communication with narcologists),[5] which is still illegally 'found', as was mentioned by PWIDs.[6] The acetic anhydride supply shrank. One of the popular methods of preparing opium is as follows. A small amount of opium is spread on a plate or pan where a few drops of acetic anhydride (which is no longer legally available for purchase) are added and dried slowly over a gas flame or heated from underneath the plate. The opium is dried on the surface, then carefully scraped off using a knife blade, which turns into powder. Then water is added (the amount of water depends on how many millilitres of the drug is desired, and then this liquid is boiled again. Lastly, the 'cigarette' sponge is thrown into a prepared solution, which is used as a filter through which the solution is sucked and injected. Some even add a few drops of blood (there is a belief among PWIDs that blood washes out poisons in the solution, and they know that acetic anhydride is poisonous). Another method of preparing opium solution for injecting is the similar. Opium is spread on a plate or pan and is dried out. When the opium is dry, it is scraped off using a knife blade, and when it is turned into powder water is added (when acetic anhydride is not available) and the mixture is boiled. As it boils the ether remains on the surface and the fluid is gently extracted via syringe and injected. Another method for preparing opium solution for injection is the following procedure, as described to me by my informants. Opium is dissolved in water on a spoon and a separately crushed tablet of Dimedrol® is added to the mixture, which is boiled over a low flame. The scum that forms on the surface is removed (because it is residue), and the rest is taken up in a syringe and injected.

---

[4] Khanka has two meanings. It refers to raw opium, but also to a homemade drug produced from tar-like opium or poppy bulbs that is in solution and injected.

[5] Interview, October 2010.

[6] Interviews, November 2010.

4.4.2 Heroin Sniffing

Heroin sniffers also mentioned to me that the first time they sniffed heroin they felt really bad and vomited. To prevent vomiting and nausea, all PWIDs said they took Dimedrol® tablets to prevent all the negative side effects, but after their body got used to it, they stopped taking Dimedrol®. The shift from sniffing to smoking and then later to injecting was remembered differently by different PWIDs. Most of the respondents who started out sniffing heroin didn't believe that that method of consuming the drug would lead to dependency. Another respondent, Bahtier (male, 33), remembered that he stopped sniffing heroin because of the damage it caused to his nasal cavity.

4.4.3 Heroin Smoking Patterns

Most of the drug users I interviewed mentioned the same pattern of smoking heroin using foil. You take the cap from a flask and wrap foil around in the shape of a spoon. The heroin is then placed in the foil spoon and heated over a flame, and the smoke is inhaled using a pipe. Another way to smoke heroin was described as smoking with a plastic bottle. This method was used before 1999–2001 by the majority of drug users when heroin was freely available in markets, where it was cheaper than a bottle of vodka. More recently the latter method of smoking heroin is still practiced by more affluent PWIDs who believe that smoking heroin doesn't lead to dependence, in contrast to injecting it. There is a belief among PWIDs that 'only smoking' heroin in this way doesn't lead to dependence and the effects of the drug are not so pronounced.

Smoking heroin with *bulbulyator* (the local name for a homemade waterpipe) is another popular method of taking the drug. First two holes (using a cigarette) are made on the side of a plastic bottle. Then some sort of tube, like the ink holder in a ballpoint pen or a simple piece of paper rolled up like a pipe, is inserted into the side hole. The plastic bottle is filled with water and a hole for inhaling the heroin smoke is made slightly above the water level. Heroin is placed in foil, which is formed into a small cup. The foil is holed, so that smoke can penetrate the bottle. When you smoke heroin with a *baklajka* (plastic bottle), PWIDs explained to me, a very small amount of heroin is left in the *baklajka* and the pipe, which is scraped out and sold:

> When they smoke [heroin] with a plastic bottle a very small amount of heroin remains in the bottle and pipe, so they [PWIDs] pick out what is left. (Narcologist, November 2010, Khorezm)

4.4.4   Heroin Injecting Methods and Combination with Other Components

All drug users, both those who smoke and those who inject, abuse drugs in combination with medicines such as Dimedrol® or diphenhydramine. Diphenhydramine is an antihistamine medicine that is administered for allergies. Side effects are sleepiness and anxiolytic and antiemetic effects.

The drug consumption method varied according to period of time and the financial situation of a drug user. Earlier and traditionally, opium smoking was widespread, especially in the western part of Uzbekistan, and injection methods came later in the post-Soviet period when heroin became very popular among the youth. Injecting drugs also brought a combination of heroin with other drugs to experiment with effects, and various myths about health also contributed to the popularity of one combination over another. There are many ways to inject heroin among PWIDs. Some prefer with Dimedrol, some prefer only with water.

Dimedrol® + Heroin

Almost 95% of all drug users in this study injected heroin in combination with Dimedrol® (some PWIDs took it in tablet form, some used ampoules, some in combination of tablet and ampoule forms of Dimedrol). The information about how to dissolve and prepare heroin for injection was shared among peers, where an experienced drug user demonstrated how it was done.

Some respondents explained that they used Dimedrol® with heroin to prevent vomiting and to accelerate the effect of heroin. The injection of heroin causes severe itching of the skin, which, however, is prevented by the added Dimedrol®. Another reason for adding Dimedrol®, according to PWIDs, is an intensification of the euphoric effect of drugs (heroin, Kodatset®). These were supported by the following statements:

> If you add Dimedrol® then the kef is stronger, and the substance will not cause a reaction [allergic reaction]). (Edgor, male, age 37, January 2011)

> It prevents reactions [from heroin] and prevents vomiting. (Matkarim, male, age 45, 2011)

PWIDs pointed out that even if heroin dosage increases, the Dimedrol® doses remain the same, namely one tablet of Dimedrol® per injection or one Dimedrol® ampoule per injection. However, there are different types of Dimedrol® such as tablet form and liquid form (ampoule). As stated by my informants, the euphoria effect with the liquid form of Dimedrol® is much stronger to inject rather than with Dimedrol® tablets in combination with heroin.

All drug users who injected heroin in combination with Dimedrol® believed that over long periods of time injection of heroin in combination with Dimedrol® leads to what they call 'losing veins', 'dried out veins'. Some PWIDs who injected heroin only with water told me, 'Look at my veins, I still have good veins, and nobody would think that I am a drug user' by referring to his better veins compared to those who injected heroin with Dimedrol®).

Naftizin + Heroin

Another possible dissolving component to inject with heroin mentioned by drug users was Naftizin. Naftizin is eye drops, and its reactant is naphazoline (a 1-mL solution contains 0.005 g Naftalin nitrate). Adjuvants are boric acid and purified water. Naftizin is produced in 10-mL plastic polyethylene dropper bottles (proglaza. ru association of ophthalmologist, accessed 13.12.12). Naftizin is recommended for use against chronic conjunctivitis and allergic conjunctivitis. Naftizin is used by PWIDs to dissolve heroin, which is believed also to accelerate the effect of heroin. The possible health harm related to the use of these eye drops in large quantities in combination with heroin was impaired vision.

Usage of Naftizin was also mentioned by some PWIDs (when smoking opium) who used it initially for the contraction of eye papilla, which, according to PWIDs, widen after smoking drugs. In order to hide their widened eye papillas (it is known as the only sign for family members to detect drug users), Naftizin was used.

Diazepam and Heroin

Injecting heroin in combination with diazepam (trade names: Relanium® and Sibazon®) was mentioned by drug users from a small town. Diazepam is a tranquilizer, used for anxiety, agitation or sleep disorder. Drug users indicated that the injection of heroin together with diazepam can only be afforded by elite PWIDs. One drug user said to me, 'It's not for everybody, only those who have money can afford that' (Matkarim, male, age 45, November 2010). The price of Relanium® is equal to the price of 0.1 g heroin. The effect of combining heroin with Relanium®, as one PWID explained, is to intensify the high: 'When you inject with Relanium, it's like injecting a double dose of heroin, so you still keep your heroin dose but have double kef and no overdose, so if you want like to feel double the kef and maintain the heroin dose, then inject with Relanium; it's like buying two doses of heroin but you keep your heroin dose down' (Matkarim, male, age 45, November 2010).

Sibazon® and Relanium® are also offered together with drugs by drug barons (*baryga*) or in bazaars (local markets). One ampoule of Sibazon® costs 18,000 sum, or ~6 euros on the black market. Sibazon® and Relanium® are also used at one of the narcology centres I visited as a detoxification medication to soften withdrawal effects.

Etaminal

Etaminal is soporific medication produced as a powder and prescribed for insomnia. One PWID (Nikita, male, age 60, 2011) explained that Etaminal powder dissolves in water as a solution and can be injected as an alternative to heroin. He stated that this method is not as popular as others which are more readily available. He also noted that various methods for taking it are used, and the preferred combination depends on what's available and the price of each medicine.

Poly-Drug Use:[7] Sonat, Sedalgin, Carbamazepine, Trawmadol

Many PWIDs inject Sonata and other medications, especially in Tashkent. These medicines are used by PWIDs to hold out during heroin shortages. As participants explained, Sonata is a soporific medicine and in large doses gives a euphoric effect. The active ingredient of Sonata is zopiclone (7.5 mg).

Sedalgin is an analgesic and tranquilizer used in the treatment of migraines, headaches, and neuralgia. Sedalgin as a medicine was attractive because of its ingredients such as codeine and caffeine. Drug users explained how Sedalgin can be used. One package of Sedalgin must be pulverized and mixed with hot water. Once everything is well mixed, you wait for everything to sink and the injection is taken using a filter.

Carbamazepine is used in the treatment of epilepsy. One package of carbamazepine costs 15,000 sum (~5 euros) in drugstores. According to some PWIDs, drinking carbamazepine is very popular among young people.

Tramadol tablets (10 tablets per sheet) are prohibited but still available on the black market, where it costs 6000 sum (~2.5 euros). This medicine was also used as a substitute for heroin in the case of shortage to tide one over till heroin supplies increase. In doses of five tablets taken orally, tramadol helps to stop withdrawal symptoms. Tramadol is a narcotic analgesic used to moderate severe pain. Information and knowledge about new drugs and new tablets were obtained differently.

> Once I was sick and someone brought these tablets, I look at the instructions and saw that codeine was one of the ingredients! (Nikita, male, age 60, 2011)

Tablets of Sedalgin and katerpin are mentioned also as substances giving kef and consumed in doses of five tablets per day when other drugs are unavailable or unaffordable. According to Umid (male, age 30, 2011) and others, information regarding medications can be obtained from narcology centres where the most valuable information about drugs can be obtained.

'Knowledge' about new drugs and substitutes also comes from Russia, where most of the migrant labour from Central Asia is concentrated.

---

[7] Poly-drug use refers to the use of more than one psychoactive drug, either simultaneously or at different times.

4.4.5 Shared Drug Solutions

There is a very popular and very dangerous practice of sharing, such as by inviting other drug users to share drugs by leaving small portions of the substance in syringes. Very small portions in several syringes can add up to a full dosage. A drug user in desperate financial straits can become a *vhoj* (middleman). *Vhoj* is a nickname for a PWID who knows the *baruga* (drug dealer) well and knows where to buy heroin. The function of a middleman is to collect money from other PWIDs (who don't have access to a drug dealer, don't know where to buy heroin, or are simply afraid to be caught by police at a drug dealer's house). Middlemen try not to reveal their sources, and keeping their role as middlemen enables these drug users to earn their doses. Drug dealers also do not sell drugs to all PWIDs out of fear of being caught by the police in case a drug user is forced to betray his source in the drug trade.[8] Middlemen are usually drug users trusted by drug dealers. Each client a middleman brings drugs to must pay for his services with 1 mL heroin, which he leaves in the syringe following injection. Usually three or four PWIDs are involved, sometimes more, depending on the availability of heroin, which in the end amounts to one full dose for the middleman (*vhoj*). According to PWIDs, it is not worth it to risk one's freedom to get drugs for one client. Mobile networking and Internet access have made the services of middlemen unnecessary, and nowadays most people are connected via the Internet and networked.

Ready-made drug solutions, one of the risky behaviours for transmission of HIV and other infections through blood, were also said to be popular among drug users. The drug solutions (heroin and opium injection solutions) are prepared by drug dealers in front of drug users or prepared beforehand. The ready-made solutions can be prepared either in syringes or in a tea bowl so several drug users can just inject in the dealer's home. One bowl of drug solution is used as a common bowl to suck up the solution with syringes brought by each user or borrowed from a dealer. Such strategies were developed by drug dealers who wanted to be safe, so that drug users could leave a dealer's house without any '*veshdok*' (evidence) the police seized a user as he came out of the house. Drug users explained as well that they were also not allowed to come to a drug dealer's house with syringes in order to show that they had no intention or even knowledge about drugs in case they were caught by the police.

Marat, who is HIV-positive (male, age 37, 2011),[9] believes that he might have become infected from using a drug solution bowl placed at the door of a drug dealer where tens of drug users were crowding around to pull their doses from their syringes and some who didn't have their own syringes were also borrowing from others. Marat stated:

---

[8] Usually when police caught PWIDs, the latter were given two options: either pay for release or serve as a *podstava* (mole) for the police. It has also been said that if the police catch a PWID, they can torture the PWID until he or she '*ne podstavit drugogo*' (gives up others or names names) to the police.

[9] Interview, January 2011.

The influx of drug users was like a non-stop convoy leading to the drug dealer, and of course he doesn't care, everybody came to his place. The bowl with the drug solution was always near the door, everybody diluted his drugs, although everybody had their own syringe but would get their drugs mixed in that one bowl, and that's how it was the whole day – the one bowl served the whole convoy of drug dependents. (Marat, male, age 37, 2011)[10]

According to Nastya (female, age 27, 2011)[11] other drug dealers sold *filters*. These filters, which were used to filter the dirt out of drug solutions in a bowl, could also be sold for very small amount of money to those who couldn't afford drugs.[12]

Similar research among drug users showed (Page et al. 2006) that PWIDs were exposed to HIV infection through the use of unrinsed cookers and reused cotton, where contamination levels were high. Drug consumption in large groups under conditions of secrecy and speed where good hygiene is impossible lends itself to group infection and mass transmission of HIV and other infections transmitted by blood.

4.5   How Drug Use Started

Drug users talked about the various paths by which they came to abuse drugs. Curiosity was mentioned by most respondents: they just 'wanted to try it [heroin] and see how it felt', even though some of them were well informed about what they were getting into. Viktor (male, age 27, 2011), who was treated at a narcology centre, studied at the highest-level police academy and worked in law enforcement. He said that he just wanted to try it once to how it felt to use drugs:

I saw many drug users and I was sure that I had more willpower and would never be a *narkosha* [drug dependent] and just wanted to try it to see what made them [PWIDs] so crazy for it? What is it? And how does it feel? I just wanted to try heroin once.[13]

In most cases, curiosity was the main driver behind getting people to try drugs, coupled with a self-deluding sense of 'being different' and having stronger willpower, different spiritual values, being an athlete, or being physically stronger. Shuhrat started eating opium together with his *mahallah* friend (they were together for treatment in the narcology centre) and said that 'it was free of charge that is why we all ate opium' (male, age 23, 2011).[14] He stated that all young men in his community started to 'eat' opium which was shared for free with other 'friends' in his neighbourhood without any fear of getting hooked on drugs. They (both young men on the treatment) justified starting their drug use (despite being well informed about

---

[10] Interview, January 2011.

[11] Interview, January 2011.

[12] Filters are remnants of the injected drug recollected afterwards into this form by means of cigarette filter or cotton pads.

[13] Interview, January 2011.

[14] Interview, January 2011.

drug dependence via school and media) by saying that they weren't afraid of becoming addicted from eating opium. Most of my respondents asserted that the only way to get hooked was by liking it ('*yokdiradi*') the first time. According to Shuhrat, someone who didn't like it and got very sick (e.g. vomiting) after the first try could get hooked.

Another retired police officer (who was involved in the fight against drug trafficking) remembers that he was also invited to smoke opium (back when it was considered high-status to have opium parties) as a respected guest and afterwards he vomited really badly until he got home. After that he didn't touch it and said:

> … thank God that I didn't like it the first time; otherwise, I would also be hooked like the others. My body's reaction saved me … Some people don't like [drugs, here mentioned opium] from the very beginning, and right away they start vomiting. I didn't like it the first time. (Gafur, male, age 60, 2010)[15]

Most respondents reported that they were first introduced to drugs by close friends, such as smoking opium, was a result of being introduced to them by close friends in their *krug*[16] (circle). Most PWIDs interviewed confirmed that usually after drinking some vodka (a common alcoholic beverage to serve to show respect for a guest), it's hard to control oneself and think clearly, so you try some opium just out of curiosity.

Krug is a Russian word for a circle which is used to describe a group of people who meet regularly and do things together or socialize together. Exchange of information, material things, and other kinds of symbolic exchange within these *krugs* vary depending on the principle around which the *krug* is organized (Turaeva 2016). Drugs are also introduced at such gatherings, as a former student told me who used to study in the capital and who went to such a party and became a drug user as a result. He said:

> At parties it was necessary to serve opium. It wasn't a party without opium in our generation … parties where only vodka was served were not popular, and say take this thing away. (Edgor, male, age 39, 2011)[17]

It is important to mention that most of the respondents mentioned that their very first experience taking drugs occurred after drinking alcohol, when one has an impaired ability to assess the risk of engaging in certain behaviours. Other research (Waldorf et al. 1991) identified other functions that drugs serve for individual consumers, such as to be 'cool' or 'fashionable'.

---

[15] Interview, December 2010.

[16] By *krug* usually people mean their circle of interactions such as gathering for certain events, celebrating life events such as birthday or wedding, sometimes even just having a *krug* to get together once a month at a restaurant, for example (where people in the circle would pool their money), or someone would hold a party in their home and everyone would pitch in and give the host some money to go out and buy something nice for him-/herself. Only people with the same economic means would be part of a *krug*.

[17] Interview October 2011.

Other reasons to start consuming opium (direct quotes from the interviews) mentioned by my respondents were the following: interest, curiosity, *dolgoigrauyshiy* (prolonged potency); *arkakchilik* (being a man), so others won't think you're weak or fearful; to be part of a *krug* (close network), everyone was doing it, girls. The reasons for switching from smoking opium to injecting heroin were the following: easy to hide because there's no smell, easy to handle, fast to consume, lack of information (while being intoxicated with alcohol) about consequences, pushed by friends, opium's disappearance from the market, cheapness of heroin, popularity of heroin among the youth, everyone was doing it, stronger kef from injecting.

4.6   Heroin Replacement Is a Solution or a Trap

The previously described phenomenon, where heroin replacement was observed among drug users in Uzbekistan, might sound like an alternative to prohibited drug use, and legal drugs could be better than illegal drugs. Is that the case? As I discussed earlier, Kodatset® is officially available and sold in tablets and is designed to be taken orally, not intravenously. To accelerate the effect, drug users add Dimedrol® to a Kodatset® solution. The addition of Dimedrol® to a narcotic is a familiar practice to heroin users, and they continue this pattern when they shift to Kodatset®. As was also confirmed by my informants, the drug had severe side effects since the dosage was too high, which caused severe itching of the skin, which could be theoretically prevented by adding Dimedrol®. Another effect of adding Dimedrol®, according to some Injecting Drug Users (IDUs), is an intensification of the euphoric effect of Kodatset®.

The extremely high number of tablets (300 tablets) used for injection is 30 times higher than the recommended maximum dosage. The continuous use of this drug in such amounts leads to severe health problems, and peer sharing and promotion of the method can become a real problem among drug users. Another important risk related to this drug is that the frequency of injection also means an increasing number of needle uses. Besides individual health risks with an increasing number of injections per day, risks related to needle exchange and the use of non-sterile needles also increase. Kodatset® is not a 'gateway substance' but the cheapest available option for getting high. It attracts drug users who cannot afford heroin. Elsewhere I have analysed the alarming changing patterns of drug alternatives among drug users and Kodatset users (Turaeva & Engmann 2012).

References

Davis RB. Drug and alcohol use in the former Soviet Union: selected factors and future considerations. Int J Addict. 1994;29:303–23.

Harris M, Forseth K, Rhodes T. "It's Russian roulette": adulteration, adverse effects and drug use transitions during the 2010/2011 United Kingdom heroin shortage. Int J Drug Policy. 2015;26(1):51–8.

Kuleshov V. On the dock-A narcotics gang. *Izvestiya*. 12 Feb 1990. p. 6.

Nazpary J. Post-soviet chaos: violence and dispossession in Kazakhstan. Pluto Press; 2002.

Page JB, Shapshak P, Duran EM, Even G, Moleon-Borodowski I, Llanusa-Cestero R. Detection of HIV-1 in injection paraphernalia: risk in an era of heightened awareness. AIDS Patient Care STDs. 2006;20(8):576–85.

Renton A, Gzirishvilli D, Gotsadze G and Godinho J. Epidemics of HIV and sexually transmitted infections in Central Asia, Trends, drivers and priorities for control. International Journal of Drug Policy. 2006, 17: 494–503.

Turaeva M, Engmann B. A new pattern of drug abuse among injecting drug users in Tashkent city. Journal of substance abuse. 2012.

Turaeva R. Migration and identity in Central Asia: the Uzbek experience. New York: Routledge; 2016.

Waldorf D, Reinarman C, Murphy S. Cocaine changes. Philadelphia: Temple University Press; 1991.

Chapter 5
Socially and Culturally Embedded Drug Abuse

5.1 Social Status and Drugs

Besides health issues, there are also important social aspects of the daily lives of drug users which are important to consider to understand their way of life. In the context of a Muslim-dominated country with a long history of traditions and kinship relations, there are status systems, family traditions and other social pressures drug users have to cope with. The long history of drug consumption in the region, which assigned opium smokers the status of an elder and higher class or respected position in a community, and later, under the Soviets, he was transformed into a narcomaniac (*narkoman*), which came to be associated with negative connotations of being a parasite on society, as defined by Soviets. The Soviets also established the security-medical regimes of regulating public health, which continues to function in the post-Soviet era and which was also discussed earlier in this book. Under such conditions of continuous pressure from the state system of biopolitics on the one side and community and family pressure on the other, drug users face multiple burdens in their situation, risking their own health and putting the health of others at the same risk. To survive outside state social provisions, drug users need to have their own networks of support. One study looked at the social network and social capital of people who inject drugs (PWIDs) (Duke et al. 2009). The researchers found relationships based on reciprocity and mutual obligation and the feeling of obligation to pool money together to buy drugs aimed at (1) reducing total costs for each network member and (2) ensuring that those who were lacking funds on a given day could still have drugs. The study revealed that if one does not have his or her own syringe to inject, then other members of the network have an obligation to borrow a syringe (Duke et al. 2009: 45). My research findings also indicate similar observations among PWIDs in Uzbekistan, which sustains mutual sharing through social obligations.

The term making *gref* was mentioned by all PWIDs. According to PWIDs, *gref*(ing) refers to, for example, offering one dose, sending heroin to prison as a gift [mentioned by only one PWID], giving out cigarette filters for free, sharing a syringe if someone else doesn't have one, at least once in your life. Making *gref* at least once is what every PWID feels obligated to do by saying, 'If you end up in prison, you will be asked – Have you ever made a *gref*? … and if not, you'll have a really hard time in there' (Mansur, male, 31, 2010). To the question of how people in prison would know whether you really had made *gref*, they said, "They are very well informed and can figure it out easily' (Mansur, male, 31, 2010). Because of the great fear of being treated badly once you end up in prison, PWIDs try to make *gref* at least once to other PWIDs who ask for help.

Status and prestige are the two important values which are nurtured particularly strongly by male members of these societies. The drive to maintain both is very strong, so strong that men will risk anything for them. There is a status system among drug users with higher and lower categories, such as high-class drug users (no name), *bangi* (middle class), and the lowest class *shirovie*. I explained this system in Chap. 4 in the context of drug consumption, where patterns differ according to the status of a particular user.

Women do not participate in this system since women drug users have no status at all. Women who do not use drugs are already in minor social positions within these countries, where the rules of Islam and patriarchy dominate all spheres of these societies. Some research has questioned this minority position of women in Central Asia and the existing agency of women (Turaeva 2011, 2016, 2017). However, with the exception of entrepreneurs or older women, there are still constraints and barriers which need to be overcome by women that men don't face to the same degree. It is also widely confirmed that politics is male dominated, and government employment is not attractive in these countries. Here it is not my aim to discuss the role of women in Central Asia, which has been done by others. I would like to shed some light on the situation of women drug users and their status within the societies they live in. I will come to gender roles and gender issues in drug abuse later in this chapter.

5.2 Identity of PWIDs

All of the interviewed drug users make a lot of effort to keep their past identities by hiding their new lifestyle and their new identities as a drug user, as mentioned previously in the section on social status and drugs. This of course has costs in terms of effort, lies, pretence and psychological effects, among others. The maintenance of an old identity does not, however, last long as their dependence at one point becomes apparent, which is also one of the reasons drug users do their best to stay away from home. In the best cases, they travel to Russia to work, and in the worst and least cases, they end up working in the capital city. Physical absence is the best strategy to keep one's identity and status 'clean' within their family networks and community.

Those who do not manage to stay away from their families and neighbourhood have to find ways of secretly consuming their drugs (e.g. under bridges, garbage fields, empty houses). Secret consumption of drugs has several implications for risky behaviour, such as being confined to restricted spaces, consuming dangerous substances and other risky practices.

5.2.1   Being 'Chisty' (Clean)

Being '*chisty*' has different meanings and connotations for PWIDs. First, being '*chisty*' (not being infected with viruses) is defined and evaluated by one's appearance (clean white socks, clean clothes), which is why one tries as much as possible to care about one's appearance in clinical settings like a narcology centre in order to be included in the '*chisty*'. The exchange of information in clinical settings is very important among PWIDs. Thus, PWIDs figure out who belongs to which category and also share this information later on the outside with other PWIDs. The acceptance of 'knowing' that someone who happens to be sharing paraphernalia is '*chisty*' plays a big role. Being clean is very important when you're sharing needle and participating in various networks.

PWIDs also use this perception of 'cleanliness' to differentiate between female PWID who are in prostitution and keeping as much as possible to maintain a neat and clean appearance 'meaning' that she is 'clean' (from infectious diseases and STIs). For women this means that she will have more clients than if they weren't clean. In fact, the notion or perception of cleanness is based on a false assumption in connection with appearance and clothing.

5.3   The Power of Stereotypes and Stigma

The HIV epidemic mostly affects socially excluded populations such as drug users and commercial sex workers (CSWs). Post-Soviet systems and attitudes of intolerance and mindsets towards groups like PWIDs and CSWs, existing public prejudice against those whose behaviour is seen as 'anti-social' or 'immoral' force already marginalized groups to continue in their risky behaviour. So they are trapped in a vicious circle.

> The dominant opinion shared by the majority is that HIV/AIDS and as well drug dependence have roots in dissoluteness and go against 'Uzbek mentality' (*uzbekchilik*) and traditions. Becker in his book Outsiders (1963) indicated 'The deviant is one to whom that label has successfully been applied; deviant behaviour is behaviour that people so label.' (Becker 1963: 9)

Male drug users would rather steal from distant neighbourhoods to keep their practices secret and keep their status within their own communities. In small cities such strategies cannot be applied, for example in a small town, everybody more or less knows each other, who is who, who is whose son/daughter. Social pressures and other obligations push drug users often to unsafe or risky practices. Social status is not retained only by individuals but is also of interest to families and kinship groups. Such practices of keeping a family member at home in secret was also practiced by many families.

Besides social pressure and stigma within one's neighbourhood and families, the major problem is harassment by the police. Many of my respondents were concerned about police who identify drug users by looking at the skin on people's hands looking for injections marks. One of the respondents stated:

> They [police] just catch you and check your hands to find any trace of injections, so if they find any, they can easily hang on you any ongoing case of stealing and beat you, so if you are caught you have to pay a bribe to get away from them. (Oybek (2), male, age 35, 2010)[1]

The methods for getting rid of injection traces on the skin include applying alcohol or injecting in hidden parts of the body. Drug users caught by the police must buy their freedom by paying bribes. Drug users without the means to buy their freedom face abuse and violence and are mostly used as scapegoats to close open criminal cases (*prishit delo*).[2] Another respondent stated:

> If there is crime in our neighbourhood, the first person who will be brought in for questioning to the police is me [PWIDs, those who were discharged from prison]. (Hakim, male, age 33, 2011)[3]

Most of my respondents bought their freedom when they were detained by the police. Another respondent observed a change in the reporting system of police on drug users between Soviet and post-Soviet times and stated:

> Before [in Soviet times] they did not consider drug abuse and did not report it so as to paint a rosier statistical picture of a region, but now the more drug users are caught, the better it is for a policeman's career. (Marat, male, age 37, 2011)

It is obvious that the police target primarily drug users in order to fill drug arrest quotas.

5.3.1   Home Methods of Treating Drug Dependence

Ne vynosi musor iz doma (don't air your dirty laundry) is a popular proverb which is very important in Uzbek society. This proverb is very important since it means that anything bad within a family should be kept secret from others in order to maintain the family's social status within the community. For instance, families with male drug-using members will try to treat him at home. There are cases where families installed a cage in their home to lock up their drug user members to force withdrawal. Elite members of society also treat family members (sons, daughters,

---

[1] Interview, December 2010.

[2] *Prishit delo* is from Russian and means 'to sew a case', that is to accuse someone of a crime which was open and not resolved, which is a common police tactic throughout the post-Soviet space.

[3] Interview, January 2011.

husbands) at home and avoid publicity to prevent damage to their reputation. They would hire medical doctors for USD 300–500 to treat their drug-dependent children at home by 'purging his blood' of heroin with all kinds of infusions and subjecting them to supervision by a nurse. These practices led to the internalization of drug abuse problems within families and kinship groups. Home methods of confining drug users in cages were not successful; drug users managed to escape from their home prison or move out. One story of caging up a family member in the living room by the parents is telling. The father of a drug user, after finding out that his son was a drug dependent, ordered that a metal cage be built in the middle of the living room and imprisoned his son there for several months. Finally, when the family left the house the drug user son managed to get his hands on the landline telephone to make an emergency call to his 'friends' and asked them to help him escape. During the escape the men took everything that moved out of the house to sell. The parents were surprised to come back to an empty house. If a parent has access to a prison cell, he might use it to treat his child's drug dependence. Other parents believe that harsh beatings and corporal punishment help to 'bring their children to their senses'.

Drug users whose identity was disclosed to their communities no longer cared very much about their status and even acted contrary to socially accepted norms. Many of the respondents indicated that many or most PWIDs try their best to move out of their neighbourhood and town and announce that they have 'gone to Russia' to keep their lifestyle hidden.[4]

5.3.2   Health Problems

The rate of HIV infection is unknown since people avoid such places as AIDS centres, as I discussed earlier in the book. Among known cases, the infection is more prevalent among male than female drug users, which can be explained either through the migratory behaviour of men or HIV test requirements for an official marriage (men tend remarry more often than women).

The type of hepatitis drug users were infected with was not known even when they tested positive since no distinction in types of hepatitis was made in places where drug users were tested. UNODC (2006) in Uzbekistan, which surveyed 1000 drug users, found that among the interviewed, 18% of drug users had hepatitis B, 12% had hepatitis C, 9% had TB, and 8% were HIV infected.

Drug users show very low health seeking behaviour due to the established biopolitics regime still operating in the Soviet style as well as the traditional cultural environment in Uzbekistan and in Central Asia in general. There is not only a negative perception about drug users among the general population, families, kinship groups and neighbourhood, but also among medical personnel as well as security

---

[4]Gone to Russia became a common phenomenon where millions from Central Asia (especially from Uzbekistan and Tajikistan) migrated to Russia since the breakup of the Soviet Union.

services who are eager to punish them (drug users, patients with HIV infection, STIs and AIDS). The latter make drug users their prey in cases where victims have something to offer (open cases for police to close, female sex service, small amounts of cash, rich families, free labour, among others). Another major reason for the low degree of health-seeking behaviour is economically driven, namely higher costs for health services despite health care being free of charge. Most of PWIDs whom I interviewed or talked to, "experimented" with their bodies in their efforts of self-treatment. What follows is an extreme example of a drug user I got to know who had to treat his dental problems himself.

Hakim is an HIV-positive, 35-year-old unmarried man who had gold crowns in his upper jaw. He went to see dentist and brought with him his collection of crowns which had fallen out of his upper teeth, and before receiving his treatment, Hakim told the doctor about his HIV infection. Hakim said that 'It was already torture to tell a dentist that I was HIV-positive.' As a result, he had to wait for a very long time, but no dentist trusted himself to deal with his dental problems. Finally, he gave up and left the dental clinic without being treated. He hesitated to go to a doctor again, and took his loose dental crowns and fixed them in his mouth with universal glue (Fig. 5.1), which bonds quickly and is sold under the local name 'moment' (glue is a prominent fast gluing substance which supposed to glue anything including metal). All know the smell and effect of the kind of glue used on shoes or other broken objects. He explained to me how he glued his crowns:

> It burned unbearably [his teeth gums] and it produced a very strange feeling in my teeth, and it was a kind of pain, or not I didn't understand really because of this shock. Then immediately I injected heroin and it turns out that after a heroin injection you don't feel anything anymore. Others could have ended up in a state of reanimation if they had done the same" concluded Hakim.[5]

Many HIV-positive PWIDs have problems with their teeth and hesitate to do anything about it because they are afraid of being rejected by health services and they want to avoid getting stigmatized. For most of them it is hard to admit being HIV-positive. To the question "Why don't you seek health care?" other PWIDs responded:

> I don't know. I try to relax and let the sickness pass. I lie down at home and let it [health problems] pass. (Ruslan, male, age 30, 2010)

Other PWIDs I interviewed outside of the clinics had a completely blue swollen hand without any sensitivity or motion. When I asked why he didn't seek medical help, he said he couldn't afford it. He worked as a loader in the bazaar where many impoverished drug users offer their services for small amounts of money. A heavy object which he was loading fell on his hand. He went 2 months with this injured hand without treatment.

Self-treatment is a common practice for avoiding extra expenses, as all my informants confirmed. Self-treatment is used not only for treating sicknesses but also for

---

[5] Interview, January 2011.

Fig. 5.1 Universal glue

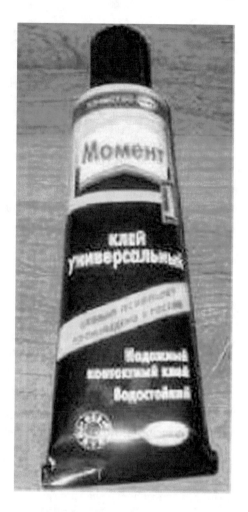

preventive measures, as I learned. Among such practices within 'preventive' measures the popular one was 'blood purging'. The procedure is performed by a nurse or a neighbour who can make infusions for small fees. Many PWIDs explained that 'cleaning blood' as a procedure aimed at reducing their drug dosage from intravenous blood injectiosn of Haemodesum-H with Analgen, Dimedrol, and glucose, which they believed made their blood more deluent/watery and, therefore, cleaner.

Another informant explained his opinion about self-treatment as follows:

> What they can advise me to do [for health problems] – I know better than doctors what I have to do for all sicknesses … these doctors with medical diplomas cannot even find your vein [for infusion] and I without any diploma can immediately get into a vein … and in our *mahalla* [local community] everybody knows that I can get to any vein, and if someone

needs an infusion [many people take prescriptions and all their medications at home] or injection, then they call me for assistance. (Rustam, male, age 50, 2011)[6]

I already explained the culture of neighbourhood nurses and self-treatment earlier in this book. Female PWIDs were all against going to dermavenereological clinics when they had STIs or other problems. They were convinced that by going to these places (such as *KojVen* dermavenereological clinic, AIDS centre) they'd have to be registered (*uchyot*). One woman believed that doctors and security workers would rather see unwanted people die than help them. That is why female PWIDs try to avoid such places and 'know themselves and what antibiotics to take'. Boltaev (2004), writing about drug users, also showed that PWIDs had been well informed about available services and treatment centres but had a negative attitude towards available programmes due to mistrust towards medical professionals. Some of his respondents stated that 'they are all connected to the police' (Boltaev 2004).

5.4 Gender and Drugs

In Central Asia women are exposed to a new risk factor: having a labour-migrant partner. Their sexually risky behaviors far from home are a well-known fact (Coffee et al. 2007). Arranged and early marriages are a tradition in Uzbekistan. Mainly girls suffer from these practices since they are given up in marriage very early against their will, which also affects their professional development and education. Due to the decrease in the male population in Uzbekistan it has become an acute issue to marry off girls. This is a result of out-migration, the drug epidemic and alcoholism, coupled with the economic collapse of the country following independence in the early 1990s. It is often the case that girls are married off to drug addicts or those who are HIV-positive (in this case of course the HIV certificates are bought) without previous knowledge. One of my informants (HIV positive) introduced me to his new wife whom he had married from a village. His first wife left him because of his drug dependence, and his family decided to find him a wife hoping that family life would keep him from abusing drugs. They found him a girl from some village because many people knew about his drug problem in the city where he lived and because it is believed that girls from villages generally don't seek divorce. It diminishes a woman's status to divorce, but if the husband is a drug addict, then it is more or less approved and they are supported by their parents. Many women whose parents are not financially well off prefer to stay with their drug-addicted husbands and at least save face by staying married. In cases where the parents of an addicted husband refuse to financially support the family of their sons or themselves are in financial trouble, it is often the case that the wives of drug addicts engage in sex work, which they are often forced into by their drug addict husbands.

---

[6] Interview, January 2011.

As a result of the financial crisis, the practice of 'transactional sex' for small gifts and money is common. Women are at risk of being infected with HIV among others and also becoming addicted to drugs. Attitudes towards drug- and alcohol-addicted persons are gender based. Men can still be accepted by their family and community, whereas women are completely rejected, and their behaviour is totally unaccepted. Men are more tolerated than women. The tolerance means receiving treatment, whether at home or in hospital, and financial help, and there is always hope for male addicts. Women are given no chance to correct their behaviour and are immediately thrown out of their safety nets, as well as from their family networks, homes and communities. The only chance at survival these women have is to leave their home-town, and this is the case in Uzbekistan. Rejection of drug- or alcohol-dependent women by their families and society limits their chances of becoming financially independent, in which case they easily fall into sex work. Discrimination of female PWIDs happens also by male PWIDs. For example, women cannot serve as middle-men, are second in line for injecting drugs or being injected by male PWIDs and they become easy targets for sexual abuse by police.

The most challenging thing is to be a female drug user in Uzbekistan and throughout Central Asia, where family status and communities are very important structures ensuring social security and daily lives. Most of the female PWID respondents started their careers as traditional singers and dancers before ending up as drug addicts. These two professions are the last resort for woman in societies like Central Asia before being forced into sex work. Dancing, singing and sex work are regarded as similar or the same in Muslim societies, where a woman is not supposed to work in entertainment or even at all. These categories of work are locally assigned to women of a lower social status and poor family background. Women from all three categories of work are not eligible to marry, which deprives these women of a future. To be a female drug user is the last thing one can be as a woman. I have already discussed the stereotypes and stigma that male drug users face in Uzbek societies, but that burden is much greater for female drug users. These women are not only ostracized from their families and neighbourhoods but also excluded from social, medical and other services. Men can be excused for making mistakes; in contrast, women are not only not forgiven but harshly punished. These women then become prey for police, criminals, male drug users and others to abuse, exploit and mistreat.

How, then, do female members of such a society end up using drugs? It generally starts when a woman goes to parties with men. *Halpas* [traditional singers] and dancers usually serve as entertainment at parties and life cycle events for both male and female audiences, which usually also ends with a smaller circle of parties for men at the end of the event, where special performances can be planned in a closed environment (Turaeva 2008). Singers and dancers suffer from the social stigma of exclusion from society (besides entertainment) and normal social lives (such as being invited as guests or being marriage candidates or simply friends). Women in Central Asia avoid being friends with or inviting singers or dancers as normal guests. On the one hand, this is very oppressive, but on the other hand it frees women from the normal obligations of female members of society (behaviour, household responsibilities serving the family, and other kinship networks). Singers and dancers are independent, make good money and are free from any socially accepted norms with some limits to keep their clients and avoid the reputation of being a 'good singer and dancer'. At the same time, dancers and singers find drug consumption very attractive. Drug consumption for women in these professions is important because it bestows power, imposes no rules, gives energy to dance till midnight, and makes it easier to relax. *Halpas* who were gradually introduced to drugs at a party or some other event might first smoke *kora dori* (opium) and come 'alive' [*halpas* usually sing late into the night] and party through the night. Most indicated that initially they liked to smoke opium before singing, which made them animated until maybe they were offered some *ok* [heroin] to smoke. One *halpa* (traditional singer), for example, became addicted to heroin:

> Heroin was cheap when I started to smoke it and I thought I could afford it with my everyday income and can stop it anytime. It was so normal to smoke *dlya nastroeniya* [to have a good mood] and being lively, singing and joking with a man, and it is my character if someone says to try something (whatever it is), I try, I don't refuse. (Rayhon (2), female, age 34, 2010)

The popularity of traditional singers means she has a good-paying job since she can earn much more money than a university professor since she is often invited to perform at an event or party. Therefore, drugs are often also a positive thing in this context by singers. For comparison, a university professor might earn at most 150 euros, whereas a singer and her crew (singer, drummer and dancer) earn at least 230 euros per evening.

Other women, particularly dancers, have expressed positive views about drug consumption as something that gives them energy and power and puts them in a mood to dance. Other women mentioned that they took drugs to ease their depression and the stress of their everyday lives.

Drug users and sex workers, unlike dancers and singers, are in a worse situation since they cannot earn a good income like singers and dancers do, particularly drug users, who will never find gainful employment and have no access to any kind of support system. All female PWIDs also do sex work as their main job and are involved in criminal activities (Rayhon, female, age 31, 2011).[7] Due to a lower educational level and because they have no access to information about risks, women drug users and sex workers are most vulnerable to health risks. A traditional singer who was being treated at narcology centre was open about her sex life without condoms, even with partner who were HIV-positive. Her idea about HIV as being equal to STIs and therefore treatable was the reason for her careless attitude towards sex.[8] She also believed in systematic self-treatment as a prophylactic measure against STIs (Rayhon (2), female, age 34, 2010).

Another category of women who were involved in drug use are the wives of drug-dependent men. This category of women ends up in sex work when normal government salaries do not pay enough to buy their husbands' drugs, not to mention

---

[7] Interview, October 2011.

[8] Interview, October 2011.

putting food on the table for their families, particularly if they have several children. This often throws the wives of drug-dependent men into prostitution since that is the only income source for women who are immobile, without social networks and left to fend for themselves.

Female drug users not only face multiple burdens of social exclusion and stigma but they are also discriminated against among their peer group of drug-using men. Female drug users are always lower in social status among drug users than men. This affects role distribution not only within the drug business but also within the practice of drug use, such as being 'second on the needle' (Harvey et al. 1998). Being second on the needle implies that when it comes to using paraphernalia to take drugs and timing, men are given priority, then women, in the context of a partner relationship, in a group, or with a drug dealer. Female PWIDs' partners (husbands) exert control 'over the logistics of injection as a natural fact of gender relations' (Bourgois et al. 2004), especially in a patriarchal society like Uzbekistan. The same holds in the intimate lives of sexual partners, where the male is seen by women as the dominant partner, such as in the case of Oybek (male, age 38).[9] Oybek is HIV-positive, is married, and was in remission from drugs (at the time of the interview) but switched to alcohol. His wife is not HIV-positive (at least according to Oybek), but they do not use condoms – for several reasons, according to Oybek, who believes that certain types of blood are resistant to any type of infection, such as his wife's. He stated:

> I had HCV before, now I am HIV-positive, and maybe my wife has this certain blood type, she is still, thank God, not infected either with HCV from me or HIV. (Oybek, male, age 38, 2010)

As for why they don't use condoms he said condoms smell of chemicals and he loses his passion when he puts a condom on. He doesn't feel anything with condoms. His wife loves him, saying, "If you die, I want to also die with you" (Oybek, male, age 38, 2010).[10]

According to one study conducted by the Ministry of Health in collaboration with the national informational analytic centre under the auspices of the Ministry of Health of Uzbekistan, in which 1000 drug users from different regions of Uzbekistan were interviewed, around 6% of female PWIDs reported that their long-term sexual partners had infected them with HIV (UNODC 2006).

References

Becker HS. Outsiders: studies in sociology of deviance. Free Press; 1963.
Boltaev A. Needs assessment on HIV and drug policy in central Asian countries, access to primary health care for drug users. Open Society Institute; 2004.

---

[9] Interview, December 2010.
[10] Interview, December 2010.

Bourgois P, Prince B, Moss A. The everyday violence of hepatitis C among young women who inject drugs in San Francisco. Hum Organ. 2004;63:253–64.

Coffee M, Lurie MN, Garnett GP. Modelling the impact of migration on the HIV epidemic in South Africa. AIDS. 2007;21:343–50.

Duke M, Li JH, Singer M. Drug use, syringe sharing, and HIV risk in the People's Republic of China. In: Pope C, White R, Malow R, editors. HIV/AIDS global frontiers in prevention/intervention. New York: Routledge; 2009.

Harvey E, Strathdee SA, Patrick DM, Ofner M, Archibald CP, Eades G, O'Shaughnessy MV. A qualitative investigation into an HIV outbreak among injection drug users in Vancouver, British Columbia. AIDS Care. 1998;10:313–21.

Turaeva R. The cultural baggage of Khorezmian identity: traditional forms of singing and dancing in Khorezm and in Tashkent. Cent Asian Surv. 2008;27(2):143–53.

Turaeva M. Feminization of trade in post-Soviet Central Asia. In: Kahlert H, Schäfer S, editors. Engendering transformation. Post-socialist experiences on work, politics and culture. Special issue of GENDER. Zeitschrift für Geschlecht, Kultur und Gesellschaft. Opladen: Budrich Verlag; 2011.

Turaeva R. *Migration and identity in Central Asia: the Uzbek experience.* New York: Routledge; 2016.

Turaeva R. Women as change agents in Muslim societies: gender and change in post-Soviet Central Asia women of Asia globalization. Development, and gender equity. London: Routledge; 2017.

UNODC. Drug Abuse in Central Asia: Trends in treatment demand, 2003–2005.Vienna: United Nations Office on Drugs and Crime: Global Assessment Programmeon Drug Abuse. 2006.

Chapter 6
HIV-Positive Drug Users: Concerns and Problems

6.1 Migration and HIV Infection

The accelerated mobility of Central Asians and increasing informalization of their societies and economies have played a role in the dynamics of the spread of HIV/ AIDS as well as drug-dependence patterns. The Russian Federation and Kazakhstan became a centre of labour migration for migrants from Kyrgyzstan, Uzbekistan and Tajikistan due to the growing gaps in wages between the migrant-hosting and migrant-sending countries. Migration mismanagement and bad migration policies exacerbated the informalization of economies and created favourable conditions for such social ills as exploitation and slavery. These have further and direct implications for the health of the general population (Turaeva 2014; Turaeva and Urinboyev 2021). The connection between migration and HIV infection is well documented (Haour-Knipe and Rector 1996). Migration may act as a bridge for the geographical seeding of HIV epidemics due to the vulnerability of migrants for various reasons such as exploitation, separation from family and partners, poor access to healthcare services, poverty and dependency on informal or criminal economies (Renton et al. 2006).

In Uzbekistan, rural areas are considered to be the most affected by poverty and economic hardship, both of which produce out-migration. As most of the country's population resides in rural areas (60%), the problems associated with rural out-migration can be said to be of national concern (UNICEF 2018). Mounier et al. (2006) argues that all risky behaviours related to social stresses are the consequences of rapid declines in economic activity and widespread poverty (which is mostly observed in rural areas) in Uzbekistan. They stated that the failure of state social security system largely contributes to the problem. In Uzbekistan, the estimated ratio of rural to urban population is 60% rural to 40% urban (UNICEF 2018). Rural areas of Uzbekistan are considered to be mostly affected by poverty and economic hardship. The economic problem after 1990 led to a drastic increase in rural out-migration. The rural-to-urban migration is mainly directed to the capital city

Tashkent, where the incidence of HIV is the highest in the country (76% of all cases). According to Mounier et al. (2006), Central Asian countries are following the same pattern of HIV epidemic as Russia and Ukraine, where HIV infection initially occurred among people who inject drugs (PWIDs) (intravenous drug user) and further spread to the general population. According to the results of the DEN (epidemiological surveillance) (2010), 69% of 1596 labour migrants had sexual contact during their work in Russia outside of marriage, 93% of them had sexual contact with sex workers, but only 33% used condoms in their last sexual contacts.

The majority of PWIDs are in Russia, where opportunities to earn an income are better. Narcology centres are reported to be overfilling in time periods when migrants return from seasonal migration (usually wintertime). Most PWIDs explained to me why, after a long period of abstinence (the duration of the abstinence varied from person to person), they took drugs again immediately upon arriving from Russia. They stated that the environment at home was inviting for using drugs again. By *environment* they meant mentality, 'friends' who were on drugs. Additionally, many of the returned migrants (including past drug users) were received at home by old friends who had parties where drugs were available.

The main outcome of the increased labour migration, especially to Russia, is the shifting trajectory of HIV transmission from parenteral to sexual (personal communication with AIDS centre representative). Structural issues such as the illegal status of migrants, unemployment, poverty and marginalization, also serve as driving factors for risk taking, namely turning to drugs and sex work as a means of coping or escape. It has been clearly shown how migration can facilitate the circulation and transfer of knowledge of methods of drug consumption from Russia to Central Asia (like the introduction of medicines, such as Naftizin, Kodatset, Sonata).

6.1.1   Condom Use by PWIDs

According to a narcologist, female drug users very rarely use condoms and mainly do not use it at all. The majority of CSWs were from rural areas. The only attitude of clients (men) is enough to avoid any trouble with clients. One of the informants, a frequent user of sex work, drew the following conclusion about sex workers: '… all prostitutes are drug dependent and all drug-dependent [women] are prostitutes, and they don't care about wearing a condom or not' (Muhtar, male, age 20, 2011).[1]

The following reasons were mentioned by male PWIDs for not using condoms when having intercourse with women outside of marriage:

- Trust (the reason of trusting those women)
- 'She is not a prostitute. She is a just divorced woman, she is not like them.' (Belief that a woman is most likely to have less sexual partners).

---

[1] Interview, January 2011.

- 'She won't betray me with other men because she knows she would be punished for that.' (Women who would be less daring to have more than one partner and loyal).
- 'She is my second wife.'(Official partners).
- 'I had one on a *permanent* basis, she isn't a prostitute but a young, divorced woman.' (This implies to the same category of women who are asumed to have not more than one partner).
- 'I pay extra for "*mama roza* (women who run brothels)" and she guarantees that women with whom I have contact are "clean".' (Professional prostitutes who are supposed to be medically checked).
- 'I don't feel anything with condom.'
- 'It is visible who is sick … I don't have relations with an unclean woman[2] [who takes good care of her body and has no illnesses].'
- 'I won't be with *cheap ones* (prostitutes).'
- 'She is very accurate [well dressed and women well cared and is presumed to have no infectious diseases as was explained in the interviews] and takes care of herself [meaning personal hygiene].'

Women (sex workers) mentioned the following reasons for not using condoms when having sex with other men:

- Trust (all)
- 'If I ask him to use a condom, he will be suspicious about me, that I had relations with other men' (ex-female PWID).
- 'I cannot insist on using a condom' (female PWID).
- 'When I am under kef I don't care, with or without' (female PWID).
- 'If I get something [meaning an infection], then I get what shall I do?" (female PWID, singer).
- 'I don't care about anything anymore' (female PWID).

Largely shared views about sexuality, family values, gender roles and other traditional attitudes towards the issues related to sexuality and safe sex are not always in agreement with established norms about healthy lifestyles and public health, and the use of contraceptives is directly related to prostitution. This implies that the discussion of contraceptives indicates one's interest in prostitution as a client or as a sex worker. Having said all this, young people without access to information rely largely on rumours and stereotypes which they learnt from their friends and the mass media (Central Asia HIV\AIDS Control Regional Strategy draft report 2009). Attitudes towards sexuality and safe sex remain little changed to the present, if posts on social media, things family and friends in the region, and what past informants tell me are any guide (2021).

---

[2] Cleanness, as defined by Uzbek men, refers to women who take care of personal hygiene (body) and are always well dressed, especially those with good *vkus* (taste) in fashion and have a great sense of style.

6.1.2   Multiple Use of Syringes

Multiple use of syringes is a big problem and widespread in poor economic contexts and where needle programmes are not very effective or trusted. Among drug users, the multiple use of syringes is very widespread, but extreme practices, such as using syringes picked out of the trash or lying on the street, are also common. Syringe disposal by clinics and others (private home nurses) is not an established practice in Uzbekistan. Used syringes are simply thrown out in the trash, and garbage cleaning system is also not well established in Uzbekistan. Hauling of trash is also done sporadically and not well organized. Street litter is common and often contains syringes.

A drug user who had found 'a sea of syringes behind a hospital' was overwhelmed by his luck. The fact that the syringes were used did not seem to bother the drug user, who frequently collected syringes from hospital trash.

To the question of whether or not they are afraid to contract an infectious disease using someone's else's syringe, most of the respondents gave answers similar to the following:

> … when you're in withdrawal, you don't care about personal health or HIV, or even about tomorrow or today; you only think about the present moment. (Mashrip, male, age 34, 2010)[3]

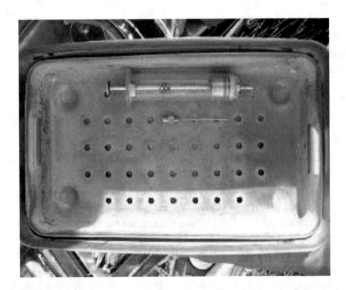

Fig. 6.1 Multiple-use syringes (these multiple-use syringes were used in Soviet Uzbekistan before disposable syringes appeared on the Uzbek market and became widely available to the general public. The multiple-use syringes were sold in complete packages with sterilizer and several needles of different sizes. Each household has its own set of syringes for family use)

---

[3] Interview, November 2010.

Others said the following:

> When you're in withdrawal, you don't think about anything else and you fear nothing – not the police or being thrown in jail or being beaten there, there is no fear of viruses (all those considerations come after the injection) – the only important thing at that moment is getting the injection and stopping the coming withdrawal symptoms. (Ruslan, male, age 30, 2010)[4]

Most post-Soviet households have multiple-use syringes (Fig. 6.1) for home use due to the frequent prescribing of medicine in the form of injections, which I described earlier. Nikita and Rustam (PWIDs over age 50), for instance, invited friends who had these syringes to their home and borrowed them for injections. They said that disposable syringes appeared later, and in their time, there were no disposable syringes available, and all households had multiple-use syringes.

Umid (male, age 30, 2011)[5] explained his sharing syringe practice which occurred due to a so-called emergency-landing situation, which he described as follows: 'we bought heroin and all in withdrawal, when you're in withdrawal, you don't care about nothing – that is called an *emergency landing*'.

Others believe that simply rinsing syringes makes them clean and safe for further use. This was often done and was believed to be safe and a way to save money, with which you could buy new syringes.

There is also a strong belief that heroin itself is a chemical and can clean even duty water and can kill all infections in a syringe if heroin is able to make even grey, dirty water crystal clean. Confirming their statement, they gave examples of where dirty water became crystal clear after being mixed with heroin.

Another common method of pooling drugs for injecting in a group was explained by Sacha (male, age 36, 2011). He said that when heroin is mixed in a bowel for a few PWIDs, it becomes stronger, but each drug user has a different dosage, e.g. one injects 2 g of heroin, another injects less, so when all of this heroin is mixed as a larger amount collected in one bowl and each pull out his own dosage into one syringe, then the drug becomes stronger and 'it feels much stronger as if you had injected a higher dose despite staying in your own dose'.

Syringes are often shared due to insufficient funds for new syringes. Ikbol (female, age 34, 2011)[6] told me that 'I was in a situation where there was a drug and no syringe'. Five PWIDs collected money (4 male and 1 female) at a narcology centre (and somehow got heroin into the centre), and there was only one syringe. She explained that there was one PWID who warned her about another PWID who was HIV-positive so that I shouldn't inject after him, to which she replied, "HIV or something else doesn't matter … I injected', and she concluded by saying 'at that time I had no idea what HIV was'.

---

[4] Interview, December 2010.

[5] Interview, January 2011.

[6] Interview, October 2011.

6.2   Networking as a Key to Survival for PWIDs?

Shirovy shirovogo vidit iz daleka (a drug addict sees another drug addict from a distance).
(Oybek (2), male, age 35, 2010)[7]

It is crucial for a drug user to be connected with other drug users forming a kind of trust networks. Drug-users, drug user-middlemen and drug dealers make up the cornerstone of these networks. These networks offer such advantages as information about safe selling points of drugs, about who a drug user can trust in terms of buying drugs, places of consumption, varieties of drugs and methods of drug use. The relations among drug users are very ambiguous and overly complex. These relations are mostly short-term, and trust is a problem there since the constellation resembles prisoner's dilemma.

On the other hand, the punishment for betrayal is severe within these networks. Betrayers (*stykach*) lose their 'reputation' within networks. If they are imprisoned, they will even be physically punished in prison. Entrance to these networks occurs through meeting at narcology centres or introduced by friends who are already members of the network.

Having other PWIDs around while injecting drugs is particularly important when there are no more veins for self-inject. In this case, assistance is needed with injecting in places that are impossible to get to. In these networks the role of middlemen (*vhoj*) is great. Usually, PWIDs in desperate financial straits become middlemen.

6.2.1   Networks as a Way of Spreading Drug Dependence

Experienced drug users as well as drug users who worked in the security services stated that the spread of drug abuse was initiated by members of the elite in Uzbekistan. It is connected to the history of drug consumption in Central Asia before Russians came to the region. In those times as well as not long ago at the peak of the drug epidemic in Khorezm it was considered to be prestigious to smoke opium and offer opium to respected guests before the Russians brought in the vodka. Although Soviets fought furiously against drugs, the tradition of smoking opium was never stopped. To this day, opium is used for party smoking among elites and is used and abused as a medicine for all kinds of ailments, including diarrhoea, pain, and others. It is often given to small children and babies to keep them calm, especially at night. All events, even small ones, especially those organized by members of the elite, have live music performed by traditional singers such as *halpas* in Khorezm with their female dancers in a band. Musicians enjoy being guests with special status and are always offered drugs. This kind of lifestyle, of parties with live music and drugs, is highly idealized, particularly by men. Many people wish to attain such a status. Those with high titles working within the security system (national security services, police and customs officers) are the ones who have direct access to drugs that they don't even have to pay for.

---

[7] Interview, December 2010.

6.3 Demography of Drug Epidemic

I have shown throughout the book drug-use patterns and their shift (drinking opium, smoking opium, injecting opium/heroin, medicine and a combination of heroin and medicine) by looking back at the history of drug consumption among local people before the Soviets came to the region where the main way of consuming opium was by drinking it. Under the strict control exercised by the Soviets after colonization of the region, drug consumption among the local population shrank but opium continued to be used to treat mild sicknesses and by elderly people as a means of keeping them productive and healthy (being healthy and physically fit was mentioned in interviews, but no research confirms their statements). After Uzbekistan gained its independence in 1991, smoking opium became very fashionable among rich people. Because of the porous borders (with Afghanistan), lack of state control (the government of Uzbekistan was not ready for independence, and the first years of independence were chaotic, and criminal gangs flourished), drug availability, the influx of drugs (from Afghanistan), the increased local cultivation of opium poppy, the cheapness of drugs (initially till 2001), the misconception among the population that opium in small quantities doesn't lead to dependence (referring to previous practices and consumption by *bangi* who could keep their dependence under control and that a small amount of opium was believed to be healthy referring tothe great scientist Avicenna). Majority of people had limited knowledge about drugs and their risks and negative consequences (financial, social, legal) which largely contributed to a mass epidemic of drug dependence in Uzbekistan in the early 1990s. Smoking opium was practiced as a recreational habit of rich people. These events with drug consumption was designating class belonging which then was aspired by those who also wanted to belong to a higher class through organising events with drug consumption parts for selected or honored guests.. These events became more and more prominent as many tried to accomodate drug consumption part of the parties which can be also observed in the mushrooming of archetectural preferences for the house constructions where a fireplace was given a special attention as a sign for belonging to a higher society namely a house which can accomodate opim smoking part of parties hosted in the same house. Furthermore, I enquired into the further questions of why there was a change in drug consumption patterns from the traditional smoking of opium to heroin if opium smoking was accomodated within the class system of local communities? This can be explained by several factors as my findings from this research indicated. First, Afghan opium cultivation declined when the Taliban banned the cultivation of opium poppy in 2000 (this needs to be reevaluated in the light of the return of the Taliban to power against the will of the West in 2021); opium poppy cultivation was reduced by 91% in 2001 (UNODC 2001) which has been also changing , and there was almost no imports of drugs to Central Asia during the period considered for this study

Another reason for the shift in drug consumption patterns among Uzbek opium users was the fact that, according to almost all drug users, opium had disappeared from the drug market completely (in 1999), and it was close to impossible to find opium, and it was expensive when it was available at all. Drug dealers said only heroin was available, not opium. It has been said that when heroin came to market, it was extremely cheap, cheaper than a bottle of vodka, as PWIDs recall as '*more* (sea)' of drugs. The price differences of drugs also determined partly the switch from opium to heroin.[8] The switch toheroin happened quickly, i.e. all ex-opium users were okay with it, i.e. one could smoke heroin everywhere and it took much less time compared to opium (which involves sitting in front of a fire and smoking the opium and drinking hot tea on top, always with friends), was not complicated, one could smoke it even at home and it has no smell. Other events, such as a terrorist attack in 1999 in Tashkent, the establishment of better border control, and a ban on the cultivation of opium poppy in 2001 by the Taliban (UNODC 2001), affected the availability of drugs in the Uzbek market (especially heroin) which was significantly reduced and thus led to an increase in the heroin price. All these factors prompted the shift in drug consumption method, for example heroin smoking slowly started to change-from smoking to injecting, i.e. a cheaper consumption method. . Economic collapse caused also mass migration out of Central Asia to Russia. Migration to Russia of local Uzbek drug users also contributed to change of drug abuse methods such as introduction of new medical substances as an alternative drug or cheaper version of drug consumption such as abusing medicines (contained Codeine) which is freely available in drugstores in large quantities (Kodatset®) or another methods such as combining heroin with other medicine to intensify the high from drugs. Another major recent shift in drug use patterns observed among Uzbek drug users was influenced greatly by economic migration to neighbouring countries like Russia and Kazakhstan. This has been explained by drug users, who changes from injecting heroin to injecting medical drugs such as Kodatset® or a combination of heroin and other medication to intensify heroin's properties and make it stronger.

Today drug dependence among young people is not as widespread as it was in the early 1990s. Based on statistical information on the demographic profiles of drug-addicted persons the population affected by drugs is ageing. This process of ageing drug users can also be easily traced in narcology centres in Uzbekistan where the average age of drug-addicted persons is 40 years. My observation is also supported by a recent report on the drug situation published by the embassy of Uzbekistan (2016), where registered PWIDS are dominated by those aged 40 to 64. Many of the drug-affected population have died from overdose, AIDS or other health complications, and many of those left the country mainly, to Russia.

6.4   Producing and Reproducing "Risks"

PWIDs produce and constantly reproduce risky behaviors depending on their 'unstable environments'[9] and on how PWIDs adapt to their 'risky' environments by producing 'risky' environment to 'others' by being the main disseminators of infectious like HIV and hepatitis.

---

[8] It has been mentioned that opium was always available and was affordable and nobody at the beginning didn't know what withdrawal is.

[9] Term environment is used in the context of political, social, legal and economic surroundings around PWIDs.

There are the following factors and aspects of drug consumption practices which lead to risky methods of drug consumption. These include constant harassment of drug users by police and absense of safe drugs and safe places for drug consumption where drug users could obtain their drugs and consume them. Constant fear from police raids leads to risky behaviors such as group injection, buying ready-made solutions from drug dealers (drug dealers started also to sell ready-made solutions so drug users would avoid being caught with drugs while exiting a dealer's house), forced injection of drugs in a drug dealer's house before leaving his place (where drugs are mixed in one bowl for countless drug users queueing up to get their share, though every drug) injecting medications like Kodatset® which requires more injections per day than heroin (three times per day) which makes one more susceptible to HIV and other blood-borne infections and sharing.

> Now basically incarcerated not for the consumption but for the distribution of drugs, so if you are caught by police, they give you an ultimatum – inform about someone who sells drugs then we let you go or have to repay oneself, , or sit in prison. And if I report anyone, there will be rumours about me and about what I did, then it will not be easy to survive, no one will trust you or sell you drugs. (Marat, male, age 37, 2011)[10]

New technologies like mobile connections (now in Uzbekistan everybody can afford to have a mobile connection) have made drug users' lives easier. Nowadays, if a drug dealer knows a user, then the user can just call a number to receive instructions on where to find the drugs they paid for (e.g. sometimes under a newspaper or in the window of a certain building entrance, or in an empty cigarette box somewhere) and one will be told on the phone where he/she may find drug and to whom money should be given first. But such techniques are used by more or less well-off drug users who can afford to have mobile phone; financially desperate drug users cannot afford to buy mobile phones; they can steal or have no connection to drug dealers.

State surveilance of unwanted groups such as drug users or sex workers, perceived high-risk groups (prisoners, PWIDs, STI patients) in the eyes of state authorities produce great reluctance to come into contact with health clinics (venereology, narcology and law enforcement) among those to whom services need to be delivered.

6.4.1 Shift from Drugs to Alcohol

A recent shift from drugs to alcohol among ex-PWIDs is becoming endemic. Changing economic and political conditions in Uzbekistan, including an economic crisis and a decrease in drug supplies, led to changing patterns of drug abuse. Furthermore, the epidemic of drug dependence taught many lessons to young people, who witnessed the tragic outcome of drug abuse of their elderly family members, friends and others in their immediate neighbourhoods. Alcohol (mainly vodka and cognac) is served in all life events and is a must at all events, big or small, and

---

[10] Interview, January 2011.

also serves as a symbol of respect to guests and a status symbol for hosts. If a host does not offer vodka at his event, he would be criticized for being greedy and for not respecting guests. One of the respondents stated that he believed that if a host, especially at a wedding, refused to serve vodka because of his religious beliefs, and even if more food is offered instead, guests would leave the wedding. He said:

> It is worth a cent all your efforts to provide with a table full of food if you will not offer vodka to guests *at least for men.* (Otabek, male, age 38, 2010)[11]

Since vodka is an inseparable part of people's everyday lives, particularly of men who spend most of their time together with their male friends or in other social events, alcohol consumptio became a serious problem in the region with its own consequences in light of economic pressures.

Due to COVID-19 pandemic-related quarantine measures, a switch was observed to alcohol consumption in combination with pharmacy drugs to enhance their effects among Uzbek PWIDs (UNODC 2020).

References

Haour-Knipe M, Rector R, editors. *Crossing borders. Migration, ethnicity and AIDS.* Taylor Francis Ltd; 1996.

Mounier S, McKee M, Atun R, Coker R. HIV/AIDS in Central Asia. In: Twigg JL, editor. *HIV/AIDS in Russia and Eurasia*, vol. 2. New York: Palgrave Macmillan; 2006.

Renton A, Gzirishvilli D, Gotsadze G, Godinho J. Epidemics of HIV and sexually transmitted infections in Central Asia, trends, drivers and priorities for control. Int J Drug Policy. 2006;17:494–503.

The Central Asia HIV\AIDS Control Regional Strategy draft report. Regional Strategy on HIV Control in Central Asia for 2009–2015. The Central Asia HIV\AIDS Control Regional Strategy report; 2009.

The Embassy of the Republic of Uzbekistan report. 2016. http://www.uzembassy.ru/05.06.17_drugs.htm.

Turaeva R. Mobile entrepreneurs in post-Soviet Central Asia. Communist Post-Communist Stud. 2014;47(1):105–14.

Turaeva R, Urinboyev R. Labour, mobility and informal practices in Russia, Central Asia and Eastern Europe: power, institutions and mobile actors in transnational space. Routledge; 2021.

UNICEF. Uzbekistan: migration profile. 2018. https://esa.un.org/miggmgprofiles/indicators/files/Uzbekistan.pdf. Accessed April 2018.

UNODC. Global illicit drug trends 2001. UNODC report. New York: United Nations Publications; 2001.

UNODC. Brief overview of COVID-19 impact on drug use situation as well as on the operations of the drug treatment services and harm reduction programmes in Central Asia. 2020. https://www.unodc.org/documents/centralasia/2020/August/3.08/COVID-19_impact_on_drug_use_in_Central_Asia_en.pdf.

---

[11] Interview, January 2010.

Chapter 7
Lessons Learned and Recommendations

In this study, I analysed the situation of drug abuse and HIV epidemics in Uzbekistan based on research conducted in 2010–2011. This research was complemented by insights continuously gained through keeping contacts via mobile applications with some of the key interview partners throughout the subsequent years, as well as updating the statistical information of the material presented in this book. Living in the region myself and travelling in the region in the 1980s and 1990s until I left to study in Germany in the early 2000s, I could offer important insights into the pressing issues that the residents of these countries faced and still face today such as public health problems, healthcare access and gender equality. The problems of drug abuse, sex work and HIV infection became more and more pressing, particularly after the end of the Soviet Union. After the end of the Soviet Union, economic devastation, opening of borders, growing insecurities and political instability have shaken already weak economies and then newly independent countries such as in Central Asia. Infrastructure decay after a long period of neglect in the late 1990s and early 2000s resulted in a dramatic situation for healthcare access, provisioning and addressing public health in general. Facilities, transportation channels, equipment, vehicles, economic conditions and personnel became worn out, outdated, broken, old or incompetent. Regaining of importance of kinship, religion and traditional values became necessary in light of the new insecurities and political and economic instability in Central Asia. This resulting mass out-migration and labour migration to Russia and neighbouring countries, which was also not organised and is still taking place chaotically and in a largely informally self-organised manner, led not only economically to remittances but also negatively in the public health situation of the sending countries in Central Asia. The alarming growth of HIV infection and escalating infection rates, other sexually transmitted infections (STIs), drug abuse, alcohol abuse and deterioration of the general health of the populations are indicators of the problems which need an urgent solution that can only be solved through collaborative efforts of Central Asia and Russia together.

M. Turaeva, *Drugs and Public Health in Post-Soviet Central Asia*,
SpringerBriefs in Public Health, https://doi.org/10.1007/978-3-031-09703-4_7

Soviet legacies of health control and health management unfortunately continue to have relevance both in direct and indirect forms, which can be analysed through carefully looking into the current practices of addressing health problems and public health management. Authoritarian approaches to health issues coupled with the challenges of traditional values and local views on practices which can be harmful to health do not contribute solutions to the problems that continue to exist in the region. The COVID-19 pandemic revealed not only the inability of local governments to address massive outbreaks of infectious diseases but also deeply seated structural and institutional deficits within the system of health care and public health management.

This book is a result of a decade of engagement with the field, with the region, as a public health expert, a native coming from the region and an activist in the field of women's empowerment and migrant support in both Uzbekistan and Germany. It is largely based on doctoral research that I conducted on drug abuse and HIV infection in Central Asia complemented by other insights I have gained throughout my active engagement with the region, the literature and the topic since the early 2000s. Since the core material presented in this book is not new (2010–2011), I complemented it with the current statistical information I collected from secondary sources. Comparison of my findings of the research, which was performed almost 10 years ago, indicate that they remain valid, due to the absence of systematic qualitative studies and largely unreliable quantitative information, and still agree with my own data from 2010 to 2011.

The study was designed to trace drug abuse and HIV infection in Central Asia, focusing on two narcology centres in Uzbekistan. The questions formulated for that study were to ask what the institutional infrastructure of managing the HIV/AIDS epidemic related to drug abuse in Uzbekistan was, how the epidemic evolved, and how it was managed (biopolitics), with a more careful look at the behavioural patterns of drug abuse and the role of these patterns in the dynamics of the epidemic. Furthermore, the study carefully analysed the link between migration and drug abuse and the factors contributing to risky behaviours of drug users.

I have demonstrated the institutional infrastructure of health management, including medical facilities, other centres funded by international organisations, security institutions and institutions within neighbourhoods, such as *mahalla* committees, which formed a control regime known as *uchyot*. I addressed the consequences of the *uchyot* regime and what it does to individuals who are already in vulnerable situations and who are left to survive on their own. The category of these unwanted people included in the system of 'wanted' or black lists are not only criminals or terrorists but also those who are discarded to fend for themselves, namely drug users, sex workers and HIV-infected men and women.

Women face even more problems and burdens, avoid any contact outside of their own communities and try to remain in the shadows. Remaining insecurely mobile and living hidden lives of drug abuse have severe epidemiological implications for all societies facing public health problems, such as Central Asia countries and Russia. The most commonly observed practices for coping with secrecy and uncertainty are either migration in order to get out of sight of local networks where hidden lives become impossible or to remain underground. The latter applies to those who cannot afford mobility – having to cope with local harsh conditions for continuing their lives of drug dependence, being HIV-positive or in sex work – whether it's in a clinic (narcology or STI clinics), at home in a neighbourhood, or on the streets harassed by police and others living inhumane lives. An inhumane orgy continues for these individuals who face violence and denial at all levels: security officials harassment within security facilities or narcologists in narcology clinics, local neighbourhood *mahallas* putting public pressure on both individuals and their families, and family members locking their sick members at home or forcing female family members into violent marriages to correct them or get rid of them.

As I outlined in this book, control regimes such as *uchyot* systems or narcology systems try their best to gain full control over their victims and oppress them to correct the unwanted behaviour. On the other hand, victims try to avoid these contacts and any encounter with these institutions. At the end of the day, as we saw even in the recent statistical data, little has been gained and no external intervention can improve the situation due to the general mismatch of local expectations at all levels.

Secrecy and fear of being found out and listed in the semi-official registers of *uchyot* are too powerful and present both within state institutions and in the minds of those affected by the problems. The notorious phrase 'na uchyote' (on the *uchyot* lists) is difficult to unroot and remains a threat for both potential categories for being listed (drug user, sex worker, infected with HIV) and those who manage those lists. These fears will only be eradicated after the whole system of *uchyot* disappears and the approach to such problems as addressed in this book changes dramatically, proving its results in practice. The European experience with addressing the problem of drug abuse, generally substance abuse, is to promote self-help groups and foster a self-help culture, where safe sex and HIV prevention can be accommodated within the Central Asian culture of mutual help and supporting the needy.

I also showed the importance of social status and gender, as well as economic situation and mobility, as determinants of behavioural patterns among drug users. Special attention was also given to female drug users, both with and without HIV infection. I detailed different life circumstances and showed the vulnerability of female people who inject drugs (PWIDs) to violence (from sexual partners, police and family members) and to stigmatization (by society and family), both of which contribute to an increased risk of exposure to HIV. Gender roles and labour distribution within both drug consumption and sex work are determined by general patriarchal social norms, which place female drug users and sex workers in the weakest economic positions, imposing the greatest labour burdens within families and heavy responsibilities and social pressures. In a patriarchal society, it is already difficult to be a woman; to be addicted to drugs in addition causes women to fall out of already limited networks of social support and solidarity (not to mention the state system of health care and social support). Misinformation held by female drugs users about infectious diseases makes them even more vulnerable to unprotected sexual practices.

Historically, the Central Asian region was known for its popular drug culture (the social status of an individual and family coincided with the serving of drugs at social events) and later for the Soviet anti-drug campaign. It is also known for the late post-Soviet replacement of marijuana with hard drugs, such as heroin. This shift has changed perceptions about drug use and drug culture. Skyrocketing numbers in heroin injection, which came with the opening of borders in the late 1990s (a decade after the fall of the Soviet Union) and mass emigration to Russia due to economic hardship, created favourable conditions for drug abuse taking on an epidemic character. Mass migration to Russia and the general collapse of healthcare systems also contributed to the HIV epidemics in the region. The coincidence of drug use and HIV infection is well known even without the additional favourable conditions for the spread of HIV caused by mass migration, seasonal migration and devastating economic conditions which make sanitary and hygienic conditions impossible to maintain not only among drug users but also in medical clinics. Even now multi-use syringes are still in use. The syringe culture in the post-Soviet countries is not new but rather a normal practice considering the popular prescription of intra-muscular injections for simple sicknesses (even colds) or for prophylactic measures (such as vitamin injections). This syringe culture led to the practice that each family had their own multi-use syringe sets, which were used for any treatment at home.

Throughout the book I have shown the links between HIV/AIDS and drug abuse. The institutional analysis of HIV/AIDS epidemics related to drug abuse and in-depth data on the behavioural patterns of drug users indicated that the institutional setting as well as the cultural background of the region influenced the behavioural patterns of drug users. As a result of societal and state pressures on drug users and HIV-infected persons, risks are created for the acceleration of the already existing risks related to drug dependence and HIV infection. The risks concern not only the infected but also their networks and the general population. Additional risks include drug injections in unsanitary conditions, the secret application of used equipment and many other behavioural patterns detailed in previous chapters.

Identity politics among drugs users was another important aspect to highlight in the book. Class consciousness and general unawareness of the consequences of drug abuse were important factors contributing to initial drug use and dependence. Initiation of drugs was connected to social events, traditions and status systems. Recruitment functioned on the basis of incentives and the necessity of maintaining one's dependence as well as an economic strategy in the situation of an economic crisis.

The status transformation of drug users has also been an important aspect in the demography of drug dependence and HIV infection. As Central Asia is a region with an long-standing tradition of opium-smoking as a component of social status, it was most vulnerable to an increase in drug dependence as drug-trafficking routes expanded in the post-Soviet period. Throughout the Soviet era, the supply of opium had been more or less secure and controlled. Soviet campaigns against drugs had, indeed, already begun to turn opium use into a social stigma. The traditional *bangi* (traditional opium smoker often elderly in a respected position) gave way in social consciousness to the *narkoman* (an anti-social addict). The Soviet era also saw the establishment of a health management regime exercising firm control over unwanted health conditions and habits. While the Soviets controlled those with 'unhealthy' habits to ensure productivity, the continued power of police-medical personnel and social workers over people with socially undesirable habits meant that these sections of the population (drug users, people infected with HIV and other unwanted health conditions, sex workers) would attempt to avoid detection, creating additional and unnecessary risks not only for themselves but also for their social networks and the general population. Younger generations and children are not immune to these risks, either.

Index

Printed in the United States
by Baker & Taylor Publisher Services